But Trish's story does not end there. The real story is how she moved through those challenges, built a sparkling character and became a supportive mother, a caring confidant to imprisoned women, a 12-step program member and a business success with a religious faith that even angry nuns couldn't ultimately shake.

Read the story of Trish's life, not to look into her struggles at a distance, but to take personally what the human spirit can do with whatever it is given. That is a blessed assurance that whatever challenges we face in our lives, we too can survive and overcome."

SAMUEL DEIBLER, B.A., B.D.

Praise for *T R I S H*

"This is truly an inspiring book! The author, by her honest sharing, gives hope to people from all walks of life. She is a power of example, demonstrating that a person can suffer from poverty, abuse, addiction, divorce and so much more, and not only survive, but use adversity as a vehicle for growth, compassion and wisdom. By overcoming addiction, the author gives others hope that they can do the same. I recommend Trish without reservation."

MIGNON LAWLESS, Ph.D.

"A hearing child with two deaf parents, an incest survivor, a parentified child and a young mother, Patricia has lived a unique life. Peer behind her inner curtain and discover a rich inner world and an enduring spirit. *TRISH* is a story of love, loss and longing told through the eyes of a girl who was forced into womanhood too early and a woman who somehow managed to retain the innocence of a girl. The author presents her experiences with such candor and strength that you immediately fall in love with her. From there, you can't help but hope she will come to love herself as unapologetically as she loves others. The impact of this beautiful book will linger long after you've turned the last page. Prepare to be changed."

DARALYSE LYONS, author, speaker, coach

"What a brave and strong woman you are! You have spoken your truth, pure and unadulterated. I am truly humbled by your straightforward portrayal of such an incredible and painfully difficult life's journey. You have reached the place of forgiveness and understanding against all odds. Your tenacious courage is palpable! This is a powerful and touching story of your journey through life, told in a most beautiful, simple way. I could hear your voice in every word. Congratulations, Trish! May God continue to hold you close to His loving and merciful heart!"

JEANNEMARIE BAKER, R.N.

"Character is not like a hothouse flower, sprung from a perfect beginning under ideal conditions. It's more like a diamond that begins as a swamp plant, is crushed into peat and coal and, after millennia of pressure and heat, emerges as a grey lump, still in need of the cutting and polishing that yields the sparkling gem.

Trish sparkles, and it's a hard-won victory in a life that has had more than its normal share of crises, challenges, struggles and losses. Byrnes squarely faces the family from which many of her challenges came. Far from the source of security and support that families must be to nurture growth and resiliency, her family of origin placed more burdens and withheld more support than any child should have to endure.

TRISH

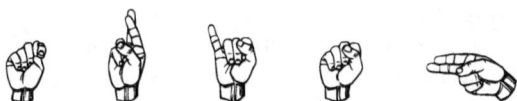

A Story of Survival and Recovery

Patricia Byrnes

Modern History Press

Ann Arbor, MI

Paperback ISBN 978-1-61599-514-1
Hardcover ISBN 978-1-61599-515-8
eBook ISBN 978-1-61599-516-5

Library of Congress Cataloging-in-Publication Data

Names: Byrnes, Patricia, 1937 February 19- author.
Title: Trish : a story of survival and recovery / Patricia Byrnes.
Description: Ann Arbor, MI : Modern History Press, [2020] |
Summary:
  "Patricia was the eldest child born into a family with a deaf
mother and father and so had to both serve as their ears and speak
for them from an early age. This additional stress, along with
childhood abuse from relatives, resulted in her acquiring substance
abuse problems as well as an eating disorder. This memoir details
her long path to recovery over a lifetime"-- Provided by publisher.
Identifiers: LCCN 2020018375 (print) | LCCN 2020018376
(ebook) | ISBN 9781615995141 (paperback) | ISBN
9781615995158 (hardcover) | ISBN 9781615995165 (epub)
Subjects: LCSH: Byrnes, Patricia, 1937 February 19- | Children of
deaf parents--New York (State)--New York--Biography. | Adult
child abuse victims--New York (State)--New York--Biography. |
Substance abuse--New York (State)--New York. | Eating
disorders--New York (State)--New York.
Classification: LCC RC569.5.C55 B97 2020   (print) | LCC
RC569.5.C55 (ebook) | DDC 362.76/4092 [B]--dc23
LC record available at https://lccn.loc.gov/2020018375
LC ebook record available at https://lccn.loc.gov/2020018376

Modern History Press   info@ModernHistoryPress.com
5145 Pontiac Trail   www.ModernHistoryPress.com
Ann Arbor, MI 48105   (USA/CAN) 888-761-6268
                              Fax 734-663-6861

Distributed by Ingram (USA/CAN), Bertram's books (UK/EU)

Dedication

I dedicate this book to my sons Zachary and Edward, each of whom has taught me more than he will ever know.

Contents

1 The Early Language of Love

I could sign before I could speak. My parents were both deaf and, as the eldest, it fell to me to be their translator. As a matter of fact, after my baby sister Barbara was born, even though I was only thirteen months old, I was in charge of signaling to my mother whenever she was crying.

Evidently, I relished this role.

You were always so responsible, Mom told me, her fingers recounting a story I had long-since memorized.

I loved hearing about the early days and how, ever since her birth, I'd protected Barbara.

I never thought to ask Mom what she'd done before I learned to sign. It never occurred to me to wonder how Mom had known if I was crying.

I was conceived in May of 1936. That August, my parents were married at the parish of St. Rose of Lima in Manhattan's Washington Heights. They were either twenty-one or twenty-two. Too young to be responsible for raising a child, too sheltered and segregated to equip me for a life lived among the hearing. Yet, it wasn't like they had a choice about becoming tied to one another. They were Catholics and I was an insurmountable obstacle. As in the case of all couples who *had* to get married, Mom and Dad's ceremony was performed by a priest in the rectory, as opposed to in the church. But, unlike so many other couples who got themselves in the family way when they were in no way prepared to be, my parents were overjoyed by my unexpected existence.

My mother, Christine Durso, had been attending New York School for the Deaf (NYSD) in New York City. My father, Joseph Byrnes, met her when he transferred there during his senior year in high school. Prior to that, he'd been at St. Joseph's School for the Deaf in the Bronx. My parents were not born deaf. Dad had spinal meningitis and Mom had some childhood illness, such as measles, which resulted in her loss of hearing.

It is not difficult to track the direction of my parents' marriage. Mom was a fiery Italian American woman and Dad was a then-typical Irish Catholic male. Filled with opinions and attitudes created during the 1920s and 30s, he had a penchant for drinking which ultimately grew into full-blown alcoholism.

As Dad's drinking accelerated, Mom grew more and more depressed. In today's world, I'm certain she'd be treated for clinical depression,

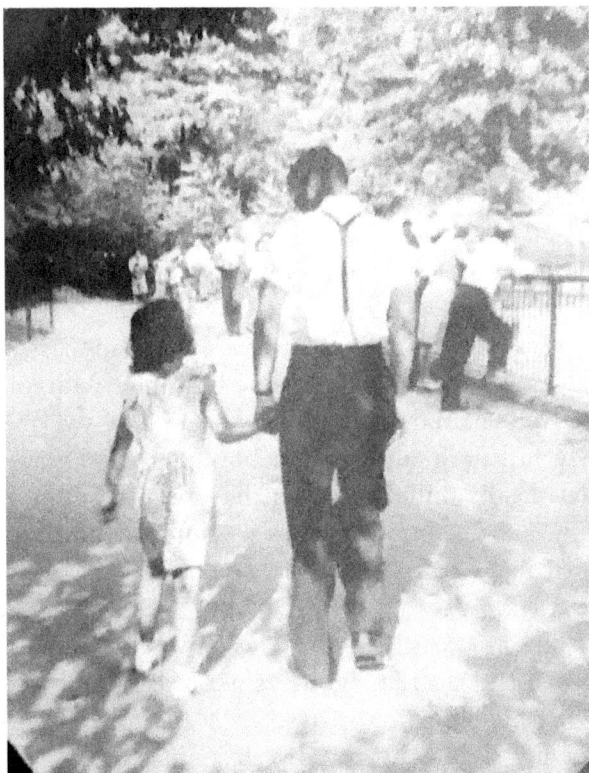

Dad and me walking, in Prospect Park, Brooklyn, NY (mid 1940s)

but in the 1930s, 40s, and 50s, we simply thought of her as "moody."

I was born on February 19th, 1937 at Lutheran Hospital in New York City's Harlem. My mother's Italian immigrant parents lived in Washington Heights, which was not far from the hospital. Dad's mother, a widow since 1929, lived in Brooklyn and Long Island, alternating between the houses of Dad's two sisters, Marie McKenna and Anna Barry. It wasn't until I got older that I started to wonder why she never came to live with us. Then, I didn't wonder.

Thirteen months after I was born, my sister Barbara came along. When I was nine, Margot arrived. Bernard was born when I was twelve. My father finally had the boy he always wanted. Dad's initial intention had been to have a son and name him Patrick, but he got me instead, which explains why I was named Patricia.

In my early years, I was always trying to prove to Dad that I was as good as any boy. I wore his old shirts, played ball, and looked out for my siblings. I saw myself as their protector and even got into a playground scuffle or two on their behalves.

Whenever we went anywhere, if we were forced to split up, I'd designate someone to act as my surrogate. Barbara and I went to summer camp for underprivileged children one year and because of our thirteen-month age difference, we were assigned to different groups.

As soon as she was given her group designation, I marched right up to another of her campmates, stared her straight in the eyes, and said, "I'm trusting you to look after my sister today."

And I meant it.

I grew up feeling shame, a silent, inward entity that governed my life. I had no friends except Barbara. We were inseparable. Sure, I had classmates at school and some age-appropriate neighbors who lived on the street where I grew up. But Barbara was the only one I thought of as a friend.

My father was brought up by an uptight, Irish Catholic mother straight from the "old country." He lived by antiquated mores and attitudes of a culture who thought girls were weaker, not as smart and just all around worth less than the male sex.

I found out many years later that my father adored his girls, but growing up I couldn't have guessed I was anything other than a disappointment.

As far as I could tell, I only ever made Dad proud in one way. I excelled at the language of sign. In this way, and in no other, I was considered exceptional. I signed so skillfully that other deaf parents used to say *I wish my kid spoke as well as Pat.*

In spite of our closeness, we were competitive. Or, rather, Barbara was competitive with me.

"I'll race you to the curb," she'd say just before taking off in a sprint."

She always won. I let her. I'd learned early on that my job was to support the ones I cared about, and I cared about Barbara so much that, even as an adult, if we were apart for longer than a few days, I felt as if a chunk of me was missing.

I can't recall how old I was when I first heard the expression "Irish twins," but I knew the feeling since the moment my sister joined me in this world. And, over seven decades later, as I began, tentatively to embark upon this memoir project, I thought about the Taiye Selasi quote:

"Being a twin, and being my sister's twin, is such a defining part of my life that I wouldn't know how to be who I am, including a writer, without that being somehow at the centre."

That's not to say Barbra and I never fought. We'd get into meaningless spats about inconsequential things. Although Mom couldn't hear us arguing, she'd sense that we were what she referred to as *rumbling* and immediately come to our shared room to intervene.

As soon as she appeared in the doorway and asked if we were fighting, we would vehemently deny it. Mom believed sisters should not fight with each other, which, I later came to realize made her a pushover where her own sisters were concerned. She actually cheated us kids of the invaluable experience of learning how to fight with and forgive each other. Even as we grew into adulthood, Barbara and I could never really get mad at one another without feeling as if we were losing some essential aspect of ourselves.

I let Barbara "win" rather than teaching her that it isn't possible to triumph all the time. Maybe, that's why she maintained her innocence and naiveté all throughout her life, whereas, even as a child, I was an adult.

When she was five or six and I was six or seven, Barbara would line up all the dolls in front of herself and I'd scoff because I was too old for dolls.

"Will you play school with me, Pat?" she'd ask.

I'd say no; she'd beg; I'd give in.

"Alright, but only if I can be Principal Sister Mathilda."

I'd retreat into the kitchen and emerge with a towel draped around my neck and a ruler clutched in my hand.

"You be Sister Barbara."

She'd eye me suspiciously. "I don't want to play that, Pat."

But I'd raise the ruler and drop it down, punishing the dolls because it was the only power I had. No matter how many times I rapped the dolls with my merciless ruler, Barbara never seemed to foresee this eventuality. She kept asking, and I kept disappointing. It was one of the few ways I allowed myself to let her down, and I only did it because I couldn't see myself as a child. I was her big sister, our parents' good girl, the eldest, the translator...

In addition to being a "spokesperson" for my parents, I was also a parentified child. In other words, I was my parents' parent...primarily my mother's.

Dad hated depending upon me, but Mom seemed perfectly comfortable using me as her voice. As she sunk deeper into depression, and Dad descended deeper into drinking, my responsibilities increased. I cared for my siblings, cooked and cleaned. I could make a bed when I was only six or seven. I started cooking when I was ten – simple things at first, boiling potatoes and spaghetti and making oatmeal and toast, which was sometimes all we had to eat. As I matured, so did my recipes. By the time I was twelve, I'd taught myself to make spaghetti sauce from scratch.

I like to think I inherited my work-ethic from Dad. I know I got my alcoholism from him.

Despite his battle with the bottle, Dad was a great worker. Deaf people don't have the usual distractions hearing people do and, therefore, his production level was very high. He worked for a printing company and, because he couldn't hear the noisy presses, so he wasn't distracted to carry out the work of lifting very heavy bales of paper onto their feeding panel. Dad was as motivated as a machine. He'd lift and lift, which was real backbreaking work. I know because pressmen were routinely getting injured on the job, and, as he got older, he had three hernia operations. But he loved his work and always felt as if it gave him a sense of purpose to conduct an honest day's labor.

In order to be productive though, Dad had to make it in to work.

I'd learned to use a payphone around the same time I learned to make a bed, and, since there was a payphone at the drugstore down the street from our apartment, Dad, hungover on a Monday morning, would give me a nickel to call his boss, Mr. Kennelly, and tell him his Uncle Joe had died and he needed to take the day off.

Unfortunately, Mr. Kennelly had a better memory than Dad gave him credit for. The second time I called to deliver the same excuse, Dad's boss replied "Uncle Joe died again, did he?"

Speechless, I hung up.

At home, I delivered the bad news. *I'm sorry, Dad. He knew I was lying.* This also fed into my feeling of shame.

Dad's boss never fired him – never even confronted him about the obvious deception. I suspect he felt sorry for a deaf guy with a deaf and "moody" wife and two kids, eventually four, to feed. Or maybe Mr. Kennelly's willingness to look the other way was purely a matter of productivity.

Dad outperformed all the other pressmen.

One day, when I was no more than ten-years-old, and Barbara was nine, we took the subway from the Heights to where Dad worked in Manhattan which, today, is Lincoln Center. Mr. Kennelly showed us around and we got to see all the tall bales of paper that Dad had to lift onto the printer. Studying the piles and reflecting on the strength he brought to his job, I was proud of Dad. I was always proud of Dad. For most of my childhood and into adolescence, he was my hero.

It was myself I blamed. Maybe, if I'd been born a boy, or if I hadn't been born at all – and Mom and Dad hadn't been forced into a mismatched marriage – he wouldn't need to drink and she wouldn't be devastated by the way her life turned out.

2

Moving on Up,
to the West Side

When I was six-years-old, we left Brooklyn and moved into Mom's parents' house on West 165th Street in Washington Heights in upper Manhattan. My grandparents owned a four-story brick building painted tan with a small garden in front and a huge backyard my grandfather used for his garden. It strikes me as dichotomous, looking back on it now, that someone whose brutality would later prove so withering could make things grow. In my mind's eye, I see Mom's dad as a destroyer; yet, he produced some good things too. He made wine (that all the adults said was pretty awful), and, from time to time, he'd acquire chickens which would produce perfectly-formed, slightly spotted eggs.

The house on West 165th Street was out of place on a street full of apartment buildings, but that was how it was with our family. We never quite fit in.

Some of the neighbors looked at us askance, but others loved our oddball house – especially

the garden. In our huge backyard my grandfather grew corn, squash, peppers, and
tomatoes. In the front, there was a smattering of
flowers and sunflowers the height of a grown
man. To this day, I'm not crazy about sunflowers.

My grandmother would sneak the neighbors
corn and tomatoes. She had to sneak. My
grandfather never would've consented to these
acts of generosity. He was a tyrant. In retrospect, it's easy to see how growing up with him
as a guardian contributed to my mother's
depression.

From the time I was about seven or eight-
years old, I did all the grocery shopping. Mom
had long-since given up.

For a while, Dad did it. On Saturdays, he'd
roll the baby carriage to the A&P and stuff it
full of ten dollars' worth of groceries. Eventually, he got tired of spending his days off
shopping and buying groceries became my job.
Because we were poor, we qualified for
donations from the church. I recall little old
ladies knocking on our door with bags full of
canned goods, but that didn't last long. Mom
eagerly took whatever handouts the volunteer
congregants were offering, but when Dad found
out what was going on behind his back, he was
so mortified he told the people who'd been
delivering free food not to come again.

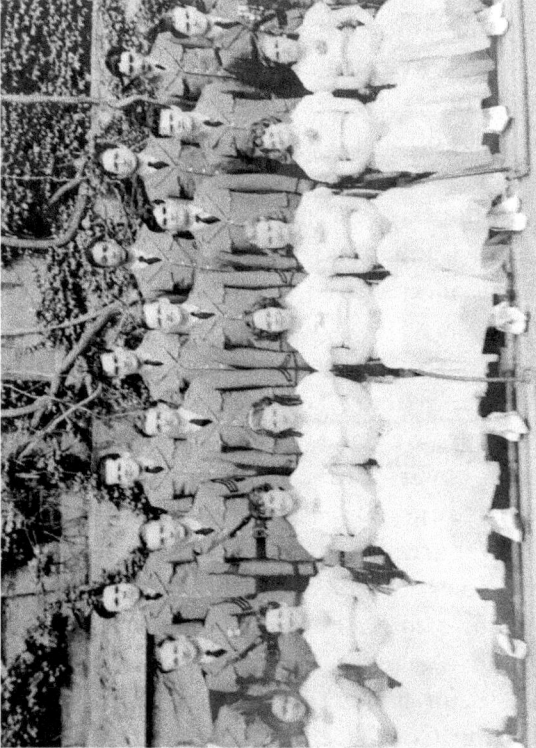

New York School for the Deaf. Graduation class of 1935
Mom is the third from left and dad is in the first row of men – second from right;

Dad was a proud man. It worried at him like hands on a wet dishtowel that he made so little that the only place our family could afford to stay was with Mom's parents.

I was never sure if Dad was ashamed of his drinking, or its consequences, but I knew that our family situation was like a kerosene stove. I would never escape the stench of it.

The odor of kerosene remains a trigger for memories of a past that shapes me in too many ways to enumerate. Our West 165th Street fourth floor apartment was heated with a kerosene stove and, as a result, everything smelled of stale, acrid gas. My grandfather was too cheap to pay for heat or hot water, which meant we had to rely on "sponge bathing." We reeked of kerosene. Bathing was a once-a-week occurrence since we did not have a bathroom. There was a closet in the hall that opened to a commode and flusher…that was our bathroom.

It was freezing, too. Aside from the stoves, there was no heat, and, since New York City ordinances forbade anyone from using a kerosene stove at night, we'd have to extinguish the stoves before going to sleep.

Thank God Barbara and I slept in the same bed. As soon as the stoves went off, we'd tuck ourselves in together and soak in the warmth of sisterhood. When we awoke in the morning, the windows would be completely covered with ice.

It wasn't until I was fourteen-years-old and we moved to the Queensboro Houses in Long Island City, just under the 59th Street Bridge, that we finally had a full-fledged bathroom. I'd stand beneath the scalding shower water, my flesh blushing a blistering pink, reveling in the luxury of hot water that I thought would wash away the memories of our old apartment.

But in Washington Heights, there was no way to scrub the memories away. There was only Barbara and me – and later Margot and Bernard – and two parents who not only couldn't hear my cries but who relied on me to make sure that they and my siblings were okay.

We lived on the top floor of the house. My mother's sister, Angelina (whom we referred to as "Aunt Juline"), lived on the third floor with her common-law husband "Uncle" Pete.

I was always leery of Pete. The gleam in his eyes seemed out of place, somehow. He was deaf too and so was Aunt Juline. My mother had two deaf siblings: Aunt Juline and Uncle Jerry. All eight of the Durso children were born with normal hearing, but three had lost their capacity to hear early in their childhoods due to measles.

"Uncle" Pete and Aunt Juline lived on the third floor with Aunt Juline's illegitimate daughter, Claire.

On each floor, next to the entrance of the apartments, was what looked like a closet with a door. Behind the door were a commode and a water tank overhead with a flusher. These were what sufficed as our bathrooms.

The first floor, which was mostly unoccupied, was a little wider than the rest. Because of this excess space, it boasted two small, dark areas. It was to one of these that "Uncle" Pete led Barbara and me after inviting us to follow him.

Would you girls like to see something? He asked us, in sign language.

Of course, at seven- and eight-years-old, we were curious.

I glanced at Barbara. When the two of us were together in the presence of adults, she was always quiet, waiting for me to take the lead.

Yes, I signed. Show us, please.

"Uncle" Pete unzipped his pants and out sprung his penis.

I was scared. I had never seen a man's penis. My brother hadn't been born yet and Dad was always fully clothed.

As soon as he got up each morning, he'd immediately get fully dressed – including shoes. He refused to spend a minute lounging around in his PJ's and disliked it intensely if anyone else was lollygagging around in theirs. That was just one of his peculiarities. One I secretly liked. We might not have had money or nice things, but we could behave as if we were respectable.

Although "Uncle" Pete was an adult and Barbara and I were merely children, I instinctively knew there was something wrong with his behavior. Barbara, too. I could feel her recoiling next to me. She didn't do anything though. As always, it would fall to me to save her. I wonder, now, if Barbara hadn't been with me that day, if more would have happened. I might not have had the courage to do anything to get out of the situation if it had been just Pete and me. I was always better at protecting Barbara than myself.

Our mother is calling us! I signed to "Uncle" Pete. We have to go!

In spite of being deaf, Mom had a voice and although outsiders couldn't interpret her various sighs and sounds, each of us knew who she was calling when she tried to get our attention. And, since Pete couldn't hear anything, he didn't know the difference. I heard though. Heard him zip up as Barbara and I hurried up the stairs.

Barbara and I never talked about that incident. I knew it had been wrong of Pete to expose himself, and I knew she knew it had been wrong, but we were being raised in an era when even children whose parents weren't deaf were conditioned to be seen and not heard. Still, after he exposed himself, we steered clear of "Uncle" Pete. I knew that if I told Dad, he'd have mortally wounded Aunt Juline's live-in boyfriend. Dad was a pugilistic person and, as much as I adored him, I knew he could be a fierce and fatal opponent. He was so strong.

Because we had no heat on the top floor, each morning, Dad had to fill the tank from a ten-gallon can for the kerosene stove. He hoisted it effortlessly. Years later, when I was twelve and he and Mom separated, he moved out and filling the tank became my job. Boy that sucker was heavy. It took every ounce of force that I could muster and at least several halting attempts, but I'd manage. I never felt sorry for myself though. I was too busy worrying about Mom, my sisters, and my brother.

Sometimes, I worried about our cousin Claire.

Like Mom, Aunt Juline had gotten pregnant out of wedlock. Unlike Mom, she hadn't gotten married in a rectory. The father of Aunt Juline's baby took off before Claire was born. Everyone said she would have married him, if he'd stayed, but they were also glad he didn't. Claire's father was African American, and in 1930s New York City although exogamy was technically legal it wasn't widely practiced.

I wasn't sure which was the source of greater shame – Claire's race or her illegitimacy. All I knew was that whenever anyone who wasn't family came to the house, Aunt Juline made her hide. Claire was three years older than I, and, although Barbara and I felt bad for her, she didn't show any signs of resentment, fear or anger.

I looked up to Claire, and I loved her. We were close, which made what later happened to her heartbreaking in so many ways.

3 Sunday Segregation

From the second floor of my grandparents' house came the wonderful aromas of Italian cooking. Grandma always made her meatballs on Saturday afternoons. Even seven decades later, I can vividly recall opening the oven where she kept a huge bowl of them and snitching one hoping it would not be missed.

Grandma made traditional meals such as maneste and beans, braccioli, and real marinara, which she prepared in a big, black iron skillet. She never invited any of us fourth floor residents to share these meals. Grandpa didn't want her to.

He was merciless in his assessment of Mom and Dad and the family they'd created. He judged us as being worth less than the rest. Worthless, in fact. And it couldn't have been purely because Mom and Dad were deaf. Mom had seven siblings, two of whom, other than herself, had also lost their hearing, and they were all included in the Sunday invitations.

Was it because my parents were poor and "sponging" off of him? Not entirely. I think Mom's dad needed someone to hate and, because Mom was never one to fight for herself, she was an easy target for his rage.

My grandfather ruled with the proverbial iron fist, and my grandmother submitted. What choice did she have? Women at the time had to be obedient. Otherwise, they'd end up abandoned, like Mom was eventually. Or with children they regretted too much to claim, like Aunt Juline.

Occasionally, Grandma would give me a plate of something delicious and whisper "Bring this upstairs to your mother," but only when my grandfather wasn't home.

Every Sunday, I'd try to think of something fun to play with Barbara. I wanted to keep her occupied. Busy. Distracted. After all, Dad would be drinking and Mom would go lay down or stare at the wall, lost in her own world. I knew why she was so upset. My aunts who didn't live with us and their kids trekked across the city to attend the church nearby our house and afterward they would all stop by for Grandmother's maneste and beans, braccioli, real marinara, and meatballs, but my mother, siblings and I were never invited. Dad either, when he lived with us.

I suspect Mom was hurt, yet she chose not to say anything. I didn't say anything either. Every Sunday, I'd focus on being the best big sister I could be, so Barbara would be spared the sadness of feeling left out. And, yet, as hard as I tried, I couldn't ever block out the upward-wafting aromas. I couldn't stop wishing we were worthy of inclusion.

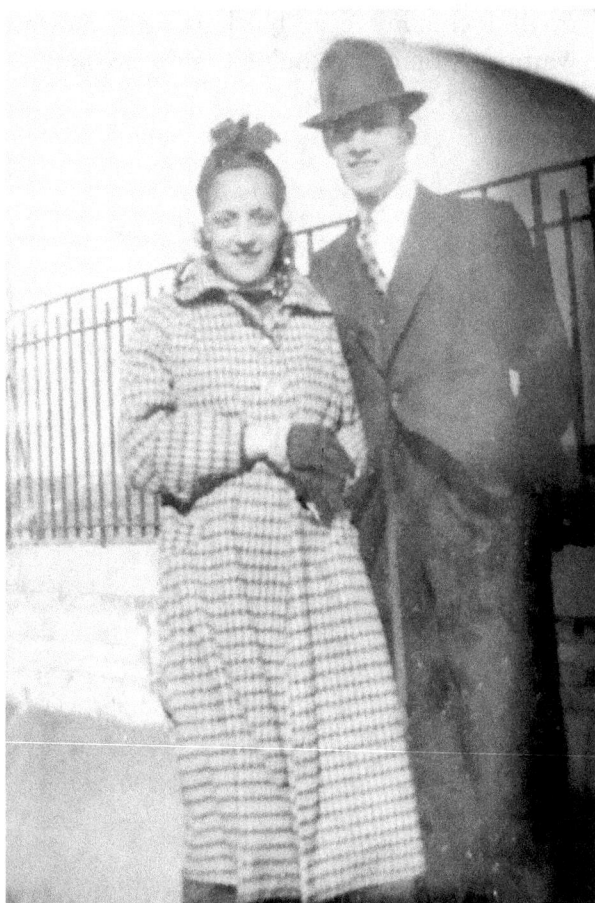

**Mom and dad right after I was born in 1937 –
in Washington Heights, New York City**

4 My Mother, My Champion

Barbara and I went to parochial school, St. Rose of Lima on West 164th Street, which was taught by Dominican nuns, a few of whom were close to senility. It was also the parish where my parents were married.

The nuns were mean. Sometimes with provocation, others not.

In my eight years at St. Rose's, I was hit twice – once, when I was in the fourth grade, for forgetting part of my homework, which earned me several whacks on the arm with Sr. Carmelita's infamous double-ruler. The second time was when I was in fifth grade. It was three o'clock. We'd just been dismissed from school for the day and were in the hallway, poised to exit the building.

As I waited for Barbara to gather her books, I popped a piece of gum in my mouth. I thought nothing of disobeying the school's anti-gum mandate since my sister and I were about to head home. But when Sr. Andrew stormed angrily down the hall, I realized my mistake.

"Miss Byrnes, where did you get that gum?" she demanded.

"At the store," I replied, at which point Sr. Andrew slapped me across my left cheek.

Since we only lived two and-a-half blocks from school, I arrived home with a handprint on my face. Mom, took one look at me and signed *Pat, where did you get that red mark on your face?*

I tried to blow it off, but she insisted on knowing and, as soon as I told her, she promptly put on her coat, leaving her apron on, and directed me to come with her to the convent, which was next to the school.

When we got there, Mom, still wearing her apron, her own cheeks aflame with rage, had me ask the nun who answered the convent door for Sr. Andrew. When the sister appeared, Mom told me to wait in the reception area until she finished visiting with the nun. The visit wasn't long. Mom got a piece of paper and a pencil from somewhere – I can no longer remember where and used the written word to express herself.

It was one of the few times that I didn't have to speak for her.

One of the few times I can remember her speaking for me.

I never knew exactly what occurred between Mom and Sr. Andrew. As was typical in our family, after it occurred, we didn't talk about it. When Mom emerged from her visit, she seized me by the arm and I scrambled to keep up with her all the way home. When we arrived, she was still hot. I listened to her banging pots and pans and although I desperately wanted to know what had occurred between her and the nun who'd hit me, I didn't want to upset her by asking any questions.

I was able to surmise that whatever she wrote was pretty confrontational, because the sister never raised a hand or yelled at me after that.

It shames me to admit what a rarity it was for me to be proud of Mom and feel as if I could trust in her protection – especially since, as I look back on it, she always thought the world of me. In contrast, Dad was my hero – tall, handsome and strong.

Sometimes, I'd look at him and think I was impossibly lucky to have the kind of dad who turned heads when he walked down the street. I didn't realize then that being handsome could be a burden, or that Mom who was objectively beautiful, couldn't rely on looks to ensure his everlasting love.

When sober, Dad was reserved and signed very little. When drunk, he was an entirely different person. Up until I was about eleven or twelve, the years were jovial and, although sometimes annoying, I didn't mind so much when his personality changed. He was still the same Dad. Only different.

Whenever he was drinking, he'd demand I give him my undivided attention. He'd sign, somewhat incoherently, and I'd find myself thinking about my classmates, whose parents talked to them verbally while they freely walked around their apartments using their ears to filter information. I had non-hearing parents. If either of them was talking, I had to look at them. So, despite wanting to avoid Dad when he was drinking, it was impossible to do anything but sit silently and stare.

Dad would repeat himself to the point of utter exasperation. His drinking impacted his dexterity, so he'd sign more slowly and "say" the same thing over and over again. In my early years, he was a weekend drinker. As time went by, his weekends started earlier and earlier until they spanned from Thursday onward and he was drunk an equal amount as sober.

It was around that time that I became terrified of him. Not the sober him. The drunk. I'd seen him hit Mom more than once when I was little.

Was that why I endured his rants? Was it fear? Obedience? A lifetime of being conditioned to be unobtrusive? It was probably all of these things. But I was also enamored of him. It wasn't until he left that I realized that part of what I loved was a lie. Dad wasn't a hero. He was a person. And, like anyone else, he'd fail, and I'd love him anyway.

When I was about twelve, after months of continual fighting, Dad and Mom separated. Or, rather, he left us. I was devastated. It felt like my safety net had been pulled out from under me. Mom was also devastated – not only by his leaving, but by the reason for it.

Although I wasn't aware of it at the time – it was yet another family secret – Dad was having an affair with Aunt Juline. I'm fairly certain I'd have figured out about them if Aunt Juline had still been living under the same roof as us, but she'd left years earlier and relocated to the Bronx.

Of all Mom's sisters, Aunt Juline was the homeliest. Perhaps that was why she tried so hard, and settled for so little, where men were concerned. Even though "Uncle" Pete had been even more inappropriate with Claire than with Barbara and me (Claire hadn't had a sister to protect her), and even though she'd have been ashamed to remain with her daughter's father, as far as I was aware, Aunt Juline never ended things with the men who came into – and later exited – her life. She waited for them to leave her. "Uncle" Pete moved out when I was about ten. Aunt Juline was ill-equipped to be alone. She'd have done anything for a tall, handsome, sign-proficient man, including stealing him from her sister.

Even before I found out about the affair, I sensed a shift in Dad. Despite his drunken irresponsibility, he'd always been a family man at heart. And he'd always taken care of us. He made somewhere between twenty and thirty dollars a week, all of which went to support Mom, my siblings and me – except for what he spent on beer and whiskey, and the money he wagered gambling. Dad wasn't a big betting man, but he'd been known to get lucky at the track and sometimes he needed to augment his earnings with his winnings. It was all always done for us.

After moving out, he changed. He was late with support money and inconsistent with his visits to us kids. The dad I'd known had been strong. Stoic. He had reluctantly allowed me to be an adult, but he'd never accepted handouts and had always done what he could to compensate for any shortcomings.

Then came Aunt Juline.

Mom's sister treated Dad as if he were incapable of doing for himself. She prepared all his meals, catered to his every whim, and even ironed his underwear and socks! Mom was never a pushover. If Dad had asked her to that, she'd have told him in no uncertain terms *Stick your socks and underwear where the sun don't shine!*

Their relationship had been based in passion and physical attraction. They were both lookers, and the sparks between them were undeniable. Aunt Juline was considerably less attractive, yet she was also considerably less likely to challenge him. And Mom could barely mother the four of us kids. Aunt Juline – inattentive though she was with Claire – mothered Dad without his even having to ask. He must've felt such relief at not having to be a grown-up all the time. And, although I'd never have admitted it to my adolescent self, I could see the lure in not having to be responsible.

When Dad left, Barbara was eleven, Margot was three, and Bernard was a newborn. Although Dad had been adamant about wanting a son, he didn't bond with Bernard at all. He was too busy building a new life with Aunt Juline. He still loved us, I felt sure. Yet, the dutiful dad I'd come to know and worship was too preoccupied with his own selfish wants to prioritize being a parent.

Eventually, he did try to establish a visitation schedule where he'd try to see us every Friday (although he missed more than a few). However, by the time we arrived at the designated bar for our weekly rendezvous, he'd be half drunk. I looked forward to these visits. Not just because Dad brought me a little bag of candy corn – he knew how much I loved them. Because it meant spending time with him.

We'd meet at the bar up the street from our house. Just Dad, Barbara and me. Margot and Bernard were too young.

I was responsible for leading the way. I'd take my thirteen-month-younger sister's hand and we'd make our way forward, not knowing what we'd find.

In the 1940s, dads didn't have interactive conversations with their daughters. So, Barbara and I would order our slices of pizza then sit, quietly in the eating area in the back, while Dad talked *at* us. He'd ask how we were doing at school, then, before we could even answer, his fingers would be on to the next subject – telling us about his life without us.

I wished Dad could visit us at home, even if he wasn't willing to move back. That way, he could see Bernard and Margot, too, and our visits could last more than a couple hours. Plus, if he saw us during the week, and not on Friday nights, he'd have been sober.

But Dad couldn't look Mom in the eyes.

Immediately after he moved out, I didn't understand why. Then, the news came out about Dad and Aunt Juline and I understood the reason for his avoidance. Still, Dad's love for us should've been enough for him to overcome both his selfishness and shame. But Aunt Juline offered him the kind of care to which he wasn't accustomed. He wanted a mother, rather than a wife, and Mom's sister was all too willing to play that role. She did everything to please and pamper Dad.

Some of his friends used to ask him why he didn't seek a divorce and he would always say, "Because I'm Catholic." But he seemed perfectly okay to sleep with another woman – his sister-in-law no less – while he was still married.

Right, Dad, because that's *okay.* I could never understand his religious rationalizations.

It took a while before everyone in the family realized what was going on with Dad and Aunt Juline. After we did, I used to get furious with Mom for never refusing her sister's company.

You shouldn't be in the same room with her! I'd rage, my hands moving rapidly as I both screamed and signed the words.

Mom would shake her head and reply "She's my sister. I can't turn her away."

Although Mom and Juline did have a couple of serious spats, Aunt Juline always knew Mom wouldn't turn her away. I knew how deep the well of sisterly love. I had Barbara. Margot too, although due to our age difference I was always more like her parent than her peer. Still, if either of my sisters had started living with my husband, I didn't think I could forgive her.

I forgave Dad, or tried to. Never mind that he'd fallen in my estimation, I'd had a lifetime of believing that the sun rose and set with him. And, also, he was the only man in my life whose kindness I could trust.

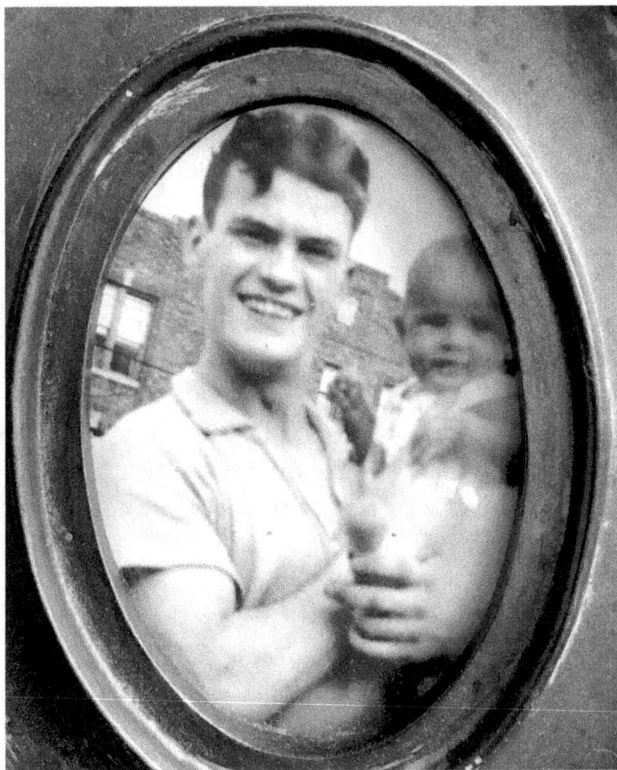

Dad holding me at six months – we lived in
Brooklyn, NY at the time.

5 Cousin Claire

It wasn't until she turned fourteen years and traveled with friends to Newport News, Virginia, that Claire experienced segregation in its truest form. Until then, even though Aunt Juline kept her hidden from inquisitive eyes, my cousin felt as if she was at least somewhat wanted. She had Barbara and me to play with and a house full of (albeit dysfunctional) family. She was sheltered, sure, but the street we lived on was, in some ways, a haven for her.

On one side of the street were Italian families – like my mother's. On the other side, all the residents were African American. Claire had kids her own age to play with. She didn't have any white friends, but it didn't seem to bother her. She was included among those whose dark skin and dark brown eyes made them understand what it was to feel as if they needed to apologize for existing. I knew that Claire had been trained to be ashamed of who she was, but so had I and I was Irish and Italian. It didn't strike me as a racial issue. It didn't strike her as one either, until the family of one of her friends invited her to go with them to Virginia.

These were people of color. They didn't know that, having been raised in our white, sheltered, half-deaf household, Claire had been sheltered in a lot of ways or that the discrimination she was used to had had nothing to do with race.

In Virginia, Claire had to ride at the back of the bus, drink from a separate water fountain and was generally kept away from the rest of the population. In Washington Heights, she'd never experienced this extreme kind of segregation. Sure, Aunt Juline had treated her like a second-class citizen, but she could convince herself that her mother's value of her was based on her illegitimate birth rather than her race.

Claire did encounter some prejudice in New York, but nothing like she endured in Virginia. After she got back, I saw that something in her had shifted and I asked her what had happened.

She looked at me, the light drained out of her previously radiant eyes, and said, "I realized, after all, that I'm a colored girl."

Anger can be insidious, especially when it becomes internalized as shame and self-blame. Shortly after her time in Virginia, Claire began what would be a thirty-year relationship with heroin. In some ways, it would prove to be the most devoted love-affair of her life. Although it may have been a volatile and excruciating bond, she held onto heroin as one of the few constants in her life.

Following in her mother's footsteps, Claire had trouble when it came to romance. She had four kids with three different men, only one of whom she actually married. And they ultimately ended up getting a divorce.

Claire would still visit us during the time she was actively using heroin. Or, rather, the person she'd become, a skeleton version of the smiling young girl I'd once adored, would visit. No longer was she overflowing with a seemingly endless capacity for forgiveness. Gone were the wide, trusting eyes. This Claire was angry, anxious, and entitled. On one visit, she stole the watch Mom and Dad had given me when I graduated St. Rose of Lima Grammar School. I was twelve when I graduated and, since I would eventually end up dropping out of high school, the watch acquired extra significance. But even if I hadn't dropped out of high school, that watch would still have meant the world to me.

It was a gift from my parents. They scrimped and saved and sacrificed to give me something. It meant I mattered. I was worthy.

When I confronted Claire, she denied what she had done. After that, I never trusted her. I loved her, always. Even felt sorry for her. But I erected walls around myself. Impenetrable walls. I wouldn't let myself believe in her again.

She trusted me. And, in her way, she tried to protect me.

When I was fifteen, Claire showed me her "works" although she didn't call the spoon, needle, and dropper that. It was only later, after I got into recovery from alcoholism and compulsive overeating, that I would be exposed to addiction terminology.

Claire had just finished shooting up when she summoned me to her and gestured to the apparatus of her self-destruction.

"Don't ever use this stuff," she warned. "And don't go around anyone who does."

I was repulsed and astonished. She seemed so blasé about showing me what she did to herself. But I took her at her word and stayed away – even from her.

What saddened me most, in retrospect, were the familial factors behind Claire's self-abuse. Yes, the cultural implications of being a person of color in a world that was designed on a foundation of white privilege generated a pain in her that, as a white woman, I will never fully know. Yet, I don't believe anymore that that was the whole picture. It wasn't even causative.

Aunt Juline's detachment from her daughter created in Claire a void that needed to be filled. Claire's mother was ashamed of Claire and, I know now, ashamed of herself. My cousin's life must have been excruciating. And then there was what our grandfather did to her. I can relate all too acutely to that. No wonder she and I both developed addictions. We were running from pain, trying to escape into pleasure. We'd grown up too fast and the only way to run from the past was to obliterate the present – her with drugs, me with alcohol and food.

Just as I eventually got into recovery, Claire eventually got clean.

When she was in her late twenties or early thirties, she was arrested for robbery and sent to a jail in Kentucky where she spent a year or two. I know they say that jail tends to make people worse, but, in Claire's case, it offered a way out. She got clean and stayed clean.

That's not to say her life was great following her release. After a few years of sobriety, she developed terminal cancer.

I learned all this by way of my sister, Barbara, who became much closer to Claire in later years. I, myself, didn't reconnect with Claire after the watch incident. I was sixteen, occupied with the demands of life, and couldn't trust her. I recalled a time when Claire, still active in her addiction, brought her oldest daughter by to visit. The little girl was the cutest. I immediately began doting on her, and so did Barbara.

"Will you watch her for a while?" Claire asked. "I have to go to the store."

She didn't come back for weeks. Someone – I can't remember who anymore – finally tracked her down, dragged her back to our place, and we returned her daughter to her. No great surprise Claire wouldn't be invested as a mother. Not with Aunt Juline for an example.

Before she died, after not having seen her mother for roughly twenty years, Claire wanted to see Aunt Juline, and reached out in an effort to connect. Aunt Juline flatly said no. Claire passed from this world never experiencing reconciliation with, or acceptance from, her mother.

As a mother myself now, Aunt Juline's disavowal of her daughter sends shivers up my spine. The child I once was isn't surprised. She recalls all too well how easily the mothers in my family found it to fail the little girls it should have been effortless for them to protect.

6 | My Other Grandmother

As dysfunctional as Mom's family was, I felt more at home with them than with my relatives on Dad's side. Dad's mother, Ellen Donohue who was from County Limerick, Ireland, was a cold person. She was universally insensitive to others, even her children and grandchildren.

Neither of my father's two sisters had any children so we four were Dad's Mom's only grandkids. Not that that made her sentimental.

One summer day, when it was still just Barbara and me, we went to our aunt's house for a visit.

"Go get me some milk from the milk crate, Pat," my grandmother ordered.

I bent down to do her bidding and the shorts I was wearing rode up. For an instant, my underwear was visible. I was maybe four or five, but she laid into me about indecent exposure and the need for modesty and said words I was far too young to understand. It wasn't my fault. I wasn't even of an age to pick out and purchase my own clothes. Yet, she criticized and shamed me, a then innocent little girl.

My grandmother terrified me. She was seventy and looked like she was 170 and had no room in her icy heart for anything other than judgment and self-satisfaction. She couldn't even care about her children, only about how their behavior impacted her own conception of herself.

Dad's mother never acknowledged his drinking until the day Aunt Rose, Mom's older sister, sat her down and informed her that her son was a "drunkard." Everyone knew Joe Byrnes had a drinking problem, Aunt Rose said.

It was true. There was no denying it. Dad's drinking got him in trouble. It even earned him a couple of nights in jail after he broke the nose of a gay man who hit on him. No charges were filed. Dad was, as were many of his generation, homophobic. And, either due to his deafness or poverty, or the social stigma of homosexuality at that time, the police felt sorry for Dad and let him go without any consequences.

After Aunt Rose's disclosure, Dad's mother couldn't hide behind her denial any more. But nor did she offer any compassion or support. She saw my father's alcohol consumption as a sign of weakness and was even more unforgiving in her assessments of our family.

I didn't have a word for her until later on in life, but I knew the feeling from as far back as I could recall. Grandma Byrnes was a hypocrite. She had no tenderness or compassion, yet she'd force my sister and me to sit with her and pray the rosary for hours. The rosary is supposed to be an invocation and a reminder of God's many mysteries, but the only thing that struck me as mysterious was how someone could be so unloving.

Grandma Byrnes died when I was thirteen. I felt no sorrow at all. Dad either. Many years later, after I had reached adulthood, my father would confess that he never loved his mother. He was sober when he said it.

Although there were many, many examples of Dad's mother shaming all of us, I recall most vividly a story my father told me when he was drinking:

Once, Pat, when I was just a teenager, my mother snooped in my wallet. She found a condom and began to berate me about it – in public. I was mortified and never forgave her.

I was horrified. Then, grateful. Then, guilt-ridden. Perhaps, if she hadn't shamed Dad about his condoms, he would've used one with Mom and I would never have existed.

My father loved his father very much.

Bernard Byrnes, who was from Roscommon, Ireland, died of cancer when my father was fourteen. I'm not so sure Dad ever got over the loss.

My father's sisters, Aunt Marie and Aunt Anna, also talked about how much they cared

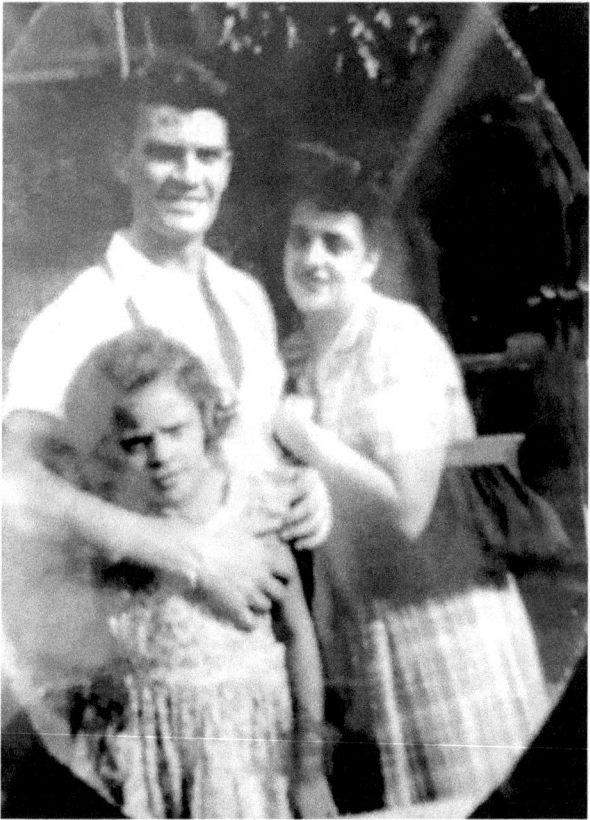

Mom, dad, and me (age 6) -
Prospect Park, Brooklyn, NY

for their dad. He was the one with the warm heart and wonderful sense of humor – ironically, an exact inversion of my mother's parents.

Mom's mother, Mary Durso was from Positano, Italy, and was a sweetheart of a woman who never complained about anything, although she had a lot to complain about living with my grandfather. She was always engrossed in doing things; a habit overdeveloped as a way of escaping from the world. Grandma was a woman of few words, but she always had a smile for me whenever she saw me. And, although she rarely stood up to the mean man she'd married, she did it once on my behalf.

When I was around nine, Barbara and I came inside on a cold winter day, and immediately encountered my grandfather. He saw my red cheeks and accused me of wearing rouge. I wasn't. The cold and wind had simply caused my face to flush, and I tried to protest that wearing makeup was something I would never have done – it was against the rules, and I obeyed rules – but he was having none of it.

"You look like a common whore!"

As he raged, my cheeks flamed even more.

I opened my mouth to protest again, but there was no need. Grandma had heard his fury and she flew out of her kitchen, spatula in hand, and scolded him into submission.

I loved her. I felt certain that, had he lived, I'd have loved my father's father just as much.

Never knowing my paternal grandfather is one of my regrets. If I simply could have met him... Then again, my own father was a fixture in my life and it wasn't until he was gone that I came to understand him.

Barbara, Margot, Bernard and I were told that our father's father died of lung cancer, but, as I got older I suspected his early demise was, at the very least, accelerated by his alcohol consumption.

When he was still alive, my grandmother hadn't been happy with her husband's drinking. Although she never spoke to me about it directly – barely spoke to me at all, except to order me to pray the rosary, get things for her, or mind the length of my attire – she'd make occasional comments and I'd overhear the adults talking, or oversee them signing.

My grandmother's distaste for her dead husband's drinking was probably why she insisted on remaining in denial about Dad for so many years. She didn't want to face the fact that her son had fallen victim to the same "moral failure" as his father. That was how they saw addiction at the time – not as a multi-pronged disease subject to a whole host of causal factors (genetics, mental health issues, trauma, familial dysfunction, biochemistry, and more) but as a weakness.

Alcoholics Anonymous was founded in 1935 in Akron, Ohio, but the AA Big Book, published four years later, wasn't nearly as well-

known then as it is now, and, although alcoholism was rampant, recovery wasn't prevalent.
Later, after I got over my self-pity, I'd
considered myself lucky that I had the resources
and support to recover from alcoholism and
compulsive overeating. Dad never had such lux-
uries; he died unfamiliar with the joy that comes
from a life unblunted by addiction. Still, he had
good times, just like his father before him.

Aunt Anna and Aunt Marie were fond of
telling stories that my grandfather used to tell.
Although they'd both been born and raised in
New York, they'd adopt their late father's Irish
accent and tell each story exactly as they'd
heard it.

"Ye ever heard the tale of the promised lady?
... A long, long time ago, there lived a brave
prince. He was learned and handsome and he
was kind. He had a special talent, too, but he'd
sold his soul to the Devil for it. He figgered the
Devil wouldn't never collect."

"What was the talent?"

"Well, Pat... Well, Barbara, the prince could
change his self into any shape he wanted. But
there was a price for it."

"What price?"

"If a woman should ever screech while he
was in his changed shape, he'd owe the Devil
his soul. He showed his talent all around, but
only to menfolk. Careful was he never to shape-
shift when a woman was around. But then one
day his wife said to him, 'Why don't you ever

show me this special talent a yours?' and so he did. He turned into an elegant stag and went leapin' around, then he changed into a beautiful bird and soared over head, and then he turned into a wet, slimy fish. When he'd been still a man, the prince had made her promise not to open her mouth while he was other than hisself. Yet, she saw that slippery fish and let out a startled screech and it leapt into a nearby lake and never was seen again. Poor woman sent her husband to the Devil."

I would listen attentively and wish I'd had a chance to know the man who had so impacted his children that even decades later, they wanted to emulate him.

A few months before my twelfth birthday, my mother's mother died of a stroke at the age of sixty-six. It was my first experience with death. When I heard about it, I was all alone.

I was walking up the staircase between the second and third stories and I overheard, "She's dead."

It wasn't altogether unexpected. She'd been sick for a while; yet, I recall being shocked by the finality. I sat down on the steps and wept. No one heard me. It seemed like hours before I composed myself enough to emerge, dry-eyed and stoic. I didn't show my pain. Above all was the belief that I had to take care of others, not myself.

I knew death meant losing someone forever and I felt so much affection for her that I couldn't imagine a life without my grandmother's smiles, or her meatballs.

My mother's father, Raphael Durso, was also from Positano, Italy, although he and Grandma didn't meet until after they had immigrated to America.

I had, and still have, little compassion for him. He was a cruel curmudgeon who shunned me, my sisters and my brother from the Sunday table, yet, with hindsight, I have come to identify the ingredients that contributed to the recipe of his ruthlessness.

Grandpa's mother, my great grandmother, was a domineering woman who pulled him out of school when he was only seven-years-old. The best reason we could come up with for her decision to deny her son an education was that she wanted him home with her. I now see this for what it was – emotional incest. She refused to let my grandfather out of her sight. As a little boy, he must've felt so controlled. It's little wonder he grew up desperate to exert his dominance any way he could.

Even when he became an adult, she ruled over him, insisting that she come to live with him after he got older. She was part of the package when my grandparents got married. I wanted to know how Grandma Durso (my mother's mother) felt about this, but it would be one of many questions I never had the courage to ask. I thought there'd be more time. Besides, the last thing I'd have wanted was to make Grandma Durso sad. She endured a lot in life. She'd had ten children, two of whom died, three of whom were deaf, and a despot for a husband.

Since we lived in the same house as my grandparents, a couple of months after my grandmother's death, I was asked to stay with my grandfather, an asthmatic with breathing issues, in order to administer his medicine to him. At that time, medical interventions for asthma were somewhat primitive. He had a contraption that looked like a tube. Inside of it was liquid that would be sprayed orally to open up his airways.

He maintained that he couldn't take the spray himself, but I think his attacks were convenient, their severity exaggerated. His insistence that I sleep beside him in bed, in the event of a sudden-onset episode, didn't strike me as quite right. I longed to remain beside my beloved Barbara, but Grandpa Durso had just lost his wife. He was a sick old man, and my mother's sisters Rose and Louise convinced Mom that he needed me to help him.

The first few weeks of sleeping beside him were uneventful. Then one night, the lights went on unexpectedly. I was a sound sleeper so I hadn't heard him slide out of bed to turn on the lights, but I felt the harsh glare in my face. As I felt my tiny twelve-year-old body being slid to the edge of the bed, I pretended to be fast asleep. My heart pounded. I felt my nightgown rise up and my underwear slide off, but I was too scared to struggle or protest. When he penetrated me, a sharp pain went through my whole body.

I don't recall if I went back to sleep. I tried to. It was the middle of the night, after all. Yet, I am certain that after that incident I knew immediately that I would never be the same.

I don't recall how long these unwanted sexual intrusions went on, but I am all too aware of their enduring impact. I started to do poorly in school, and began the practice of staring into space. Feeling removed from my body was my only way to escape. I'd lose track of time. I'd lose myself.

Eventually, I told my mother I didn't want to sleep with Grandpa Durso anymore. Despite my fear that she'd force me to continue playing nursemaid to my abuser, she allowed me to return to the bed Barbara and I shared.

But even after he no longer had unrestricted nightly access to me, I wasn't free of him. There were a handful of occasions during which he enticed me to join him in private. Each time, he said he was going to make me "feel good." This happened at a time when Dad had left. We were all depressed, but I felt particularly abandoned by him. Anything that would help me feel better was almost welcome.

I expected my grandfather to protest when I stopped joining him in bed at night, but he let the situation go. I wasn't sure why. I wouldn't have blackmailed him. Not the way he blackmailed me, giving me money in exchange for my silence when, even without inducement, I never would have told. I thought the incest was my fault and I knew if I confessed to what was happening everyone around me would see me the way I saw myself. There was at least one person I wish, now, I'd shared it with: Claire. Grandfather Durso had had his way with her, too. If I had spoken about it, or if she had, maybe we both would've been spared the shame of believing we deserved what we got. Maybe, we could've found solace in each other, and in our shared experience. But I kept quiet. I didn't even tell Barbara.

As much as I blamed the face I saw every morning in the mirror, I developed a fierce hate for my grandfather. When he died in 1965, I was twenty-eight. I was pregnant with my second son, Edward, and much to the chagrin of my extended family I did not go to his funeral or wake. My mother's family thought I was being a rebel and tried to convince me to go.

Come on, Pat. He's your grandfather. Don't be so stubborn. This isn't like you...

Although I never enlightened my family about the real reason for my disavowal of the man responsible for a quarter of my genes, taking a stand gave me a small sense of satisfaction. It was the only thing at the time that I could do to get back at him.

Nevertheless, the wounds of incest remained well into adulthood. They're still with me, although I like to think they've healed enough that their scars are almost imperceptible.

It was not until I joined a support group for incest survivors when I was fifty-years-old that I learned about the M.O. of a pedophile. Picking on vulnerable, depressed children was a motive and I certainly fit that profile. Claire, too. I never realized how these incest experiences affected me until I started talking about them with others who'd endured similar tortures.

Until those group support sessions, the only person I ever told about the incest was my second husband, Dennis Hart, and I didn't even tell him, technically. I hinted, but I was too ashamed to tell the whole story. Dennis didn't seem especially open to hearing about it anyway, and I hadn't yet acquired a way to be open about this part of my past.

I used to say, "If I could dig up my grandfather's bones, I would burn them."

I could acknowledge the hate, but not the hurt. Eventually, I learned that my hatred toward him wasn't the defense I believed it to be. I had absorbed so much shame and self-loathing. In hating him, I hated myself.

My support group taught me that I needed to share to let go of the shame.

I knew that already from Alcoholics Anonymous and Overeaters Anonymous, but sharing about my alcoholism and food addiction had felt like child's play when compared to this deep, dark family secret. Still, I wanted to recover. I wanted to break free. So, I did what the group advised.

First, I shared the story with my son Zach and his then-wife; then, with my son Edward. After I shared about the incest with my sons, I told Barbara.

We were sitting in my kitchen when I admitted to Barbara what our grandfather had done. Imagine my shock when she looked me in the eye and said he abused her as well. I actually lost my breath to think we never once disclosed these secrets to each other. We each believed we'd been the only one. I'd never so much suspected our grandfather had molested our cousin until Barbara revealed that painful truth. Perhaps, if I'd known earlier, I might've made an effort to build more of a bridge between myself and the cousin I'd loved and lost, first to heroin, then to cancer.

I'll never know.

By then, Claire was dead.

I was fifty-one. Barbara was fifty.

I encouraged her to seek help. She made an appointment with a therapist, but never went back. It was one of those unfinished things in my sister's life which, I believe led to her cancer.

6 The Guilt of Being Gorgeous

I was smart, but I never thought I was. I never thought I was enough, period. I didn't have a patent on low self-esteem, but I was smart, pretty, and sociable and it saddens me now to think I couldn't see myself as any of those things.

It didn't help that Dad didn't believe in promoting a "swelled head" by giving his kids compliments.

I always knew Dad cared deeply for us, but he wasn't affectionate. He'd kiss us chastely on our cheeks when he got home from work, or goodbye if he was leaving, but I can't recall a single hug or snuggle. It was as if we made him uncomfortable. A few years ago, in my late seventies, I visited a priest/psychologist and told him some of my story. I thought, maybe, given his association with Catholicism and mental health, he might have some insights into why Dad was the way he was.

The priest surprised me. "You know, Pat" he said, "I'm not sure your father knew how to handle having beautiful daughters."

Beautiful? Me? I certainly saw Barbara that way, but at the time I hadn't seen myself accurately. It rang true though. Dad hadn't known how to navigate the lines of parenting girls and so, out of love, rather than rejection, he had remained respectful to the point of ridiculousness.

One example of Dad's inability to compliment happened when I was a teenager. He'd left his and Aunt Juline's apartment for a few hours to come visit us at our house. By then, the animosity between my parents had gotten marginally better. Dad no longer needed us to visit him in bars. He could look Mom in the eyes, although, for the life of me, I didn't know how.

"How do I look?" I asked, somewhat sheepishly.

I was all dressed up to go out with friends. Mom was always much more generous with her compliments and affection than Dad was. She supported me emotionally, as best she could given her battles with depression. And I have to hope her uplifting comments kept my self-esteem from being even worse than it was. Mom told me she thought I looked beautiful (to her, her children were always beautiful). But I was seeking Dad's approval. We both glanced at him.

Because deaf people aren't able to use spoken words to convey their meaning, they tend to have very exaggerated ways of emoting via gestures and facial expressions. What's more, I'd memorized every last line and wrinkle on my father's face. It was obvious from his upturned lips, slightly squinty eyes and the way his eyebrows bunched up just a little at the middle that he was proud of me and thought I looked pretty, yet he couldn't tell me directly. Instead, he told my mother to tell me I looked *very nice*.

Barbara was in the corner, sitting unobtrusively in a chair. I caught her eye and knew we were both thinking the same thing.

There is an old anecdote our Irish family members used to tell:

One fine young morning, an Irish gentleman saw a lovely young woman and thought, *Now, there's a real beauty if ever there was one*. But, instead of telling her directly, he bid her good day and instructed her to "Go home and tell your mam she made you gorgeous."

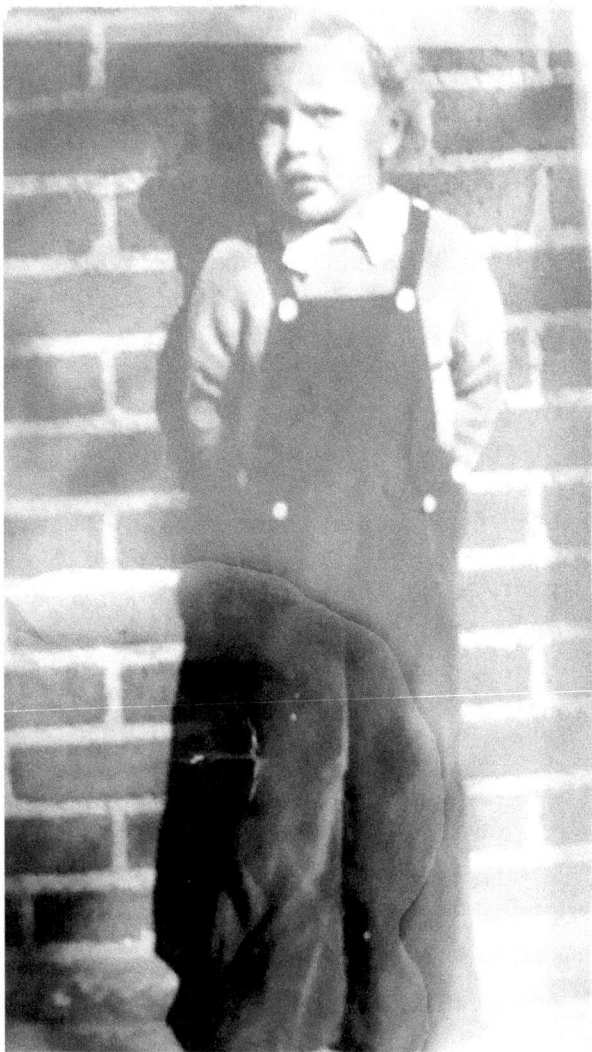

Me, alone, at two years, Brooklyn, NY

7 Secretarial Aspirations

From as far back as I could remember, I wanted to be a secretary. It struck me as the classiest job there was. What could be more glamorous than being the "woman behind the man"? This was the forties and fifties when being a woman afforded limited options. My own mother had no interests outside the home; she only ever stayed at home, with us. I didn't ever want to end up with such a narrow existence. I wanted to make an impact!

The fact that secretaries were also "servers" fed into my already existing idea of who I was supposed to be. I was the parentified child, used to taking care of, cleaning up after, and cooking for others.

It seemed only natural to leave high school at sixteen, find a job, and help support my family. There wasn't much in the way of student counseling, but, even if there had been, I wouldn't have let anyone talk me out of leaving school. Or, more accurately, a child whose life experiences had required her to grow up too early.

The teachers at Julia Richman High School tried to dissuade me from giving up on my education. I didn't care about their opinions, but I did care about Dad's. He was heartbroken that I was leaving school. Mom was barely making ends meet, however, and he was erratic with his support. Besides, I was consumed with the idea of going out into the working world. I was sixteen going on twenty-six and I felt I had something to prove.

And prove myself I did.

My first job was working in the Records Room of Columbia Presbyterian Medical Center in Washington Heights. Back then, there were no computers, only paper charts. We workers were tasked with filing the charts, pulling patient files, bringing them to the rooms for doctors to use, and then returning them where they belonged.

My favorite part was carrying charts to their respective units. I got to see a lot of people, sick people to whom I could deliver not only a file, but a smile. Not all of the patients were sick. In the pediatric wing of the hospital, I'd get to see all the babies. I loved my role as a records clerk.

I still had my eye on being a secretary. At night, after working an eight-hour day at the hospital, I would practice writing shorthand while listening to the radio. I'd kept my Pitman

Shorthand book from school and I painstak-
ingly reviewed all the lessons I learned.

During the summer of my sixteenth year
(1953), when I'd already dropped out of school,
but was far less adult than I believed myself to
be, I met my first boyfriend, Bert Young. Bert's
brother, Joe, was married to my cousin, Rose
(Mom's sister's daughter). I became immediately
infatuated with Bert, although at the time I
called it love.

I hoped he might "love" me in return, but his
only goal was to "Put me down" – a local New
York City expression for having sex. Although I
didn't know until much later – after it was too
late – Bert had made a bet with some of the
other boys in the neighborhood. To them, I was
the picture of a good Catholic girl and Bert
made it his quest to deflower me so he could
brag about it. I'm not sure if the bet involved
money or if it was just boasting rights he
wanted.

All I knew was that I'd already been
deflowered, a fact about which I regularly
agonized. I thought I was going to hell. Part of
me wanted to do all I could to earn forgiveness
and live the life of a saint. Another part felt as if
I'd already sinned by "being with" my grandfather and was convinced I'd never be able to
atone. My first experience with consensual sex
should've been precious, yet I felt as if I were a
sinner.

Nevertheless, in spite of my harsh and unwarranted self-assessment, I had internalized the "good girl" values with which I'd been indoctrinated. All those years with the nuns, and all those lectures from the women in my family – some of whom had been "put down" early on and often – instilled in me the belief that sex was dirty. I refused Bert's advances. He threatened to leave me. I was faced with a decision. Not the decision that occurs to my adult mind now as I look back at my sixteen-year-old self (Succumb to Bert's advances or refuse?), but the decision the young, in-love, shame-filled me thought she had. I was torn between whether or not to tell Bert I wasn't a virgin.

I knew that if we had sex, he'd know he hadn't been the first. My hymen was gone, and with it my innocence.

My hands were shaking when I told Bert that I wasn't a virgin. I didn't tell him that my virginity had been stolen, rather than offered. But it wouldn't have mattered. He was an eighteen-year-old, full of hormones. He didn't ask me a single question. All he said was, "So. I don't care."

After that, Bert and I had sex a few times in the back of his Chevy. Then, because I was no longer a challenge – he'd gotten what he wanted – he ended it. He didn't come right out and tell me, either. He simply stopped calling and eventually I put two and two together. I was heartbroken. I was just a teenager and I'd thought sex meant love.

In the fall of 1953, I missed my period. I didn't say anything to my mother. I simply did as many sit-ups as I could, trying to coax my period into arriving like Bert had coaxed me into his backseat.

Two more periods were missed.

After three months, I knew I couldn't stay silent.

But how could I tell my parents? Or my siblings? Or anyone?

I told Claire. Never mind that, by that point, I had already learned to untrust her. She knew the feeling of being a mistake. I felt certain she wouldn't judge me.

Since she was also able to sign, Claire went to Dad and Mom, without me, and told them I was pregnant. I agonized the entire time that she was gone. Would they judge me as harshly as I judged myself? Would they disown me?

Contrary to my fears, my parents never chastised me.

In those days, girls either gave their babies up for adoption, or got married. Abortion was not legal, and I would not have had one anyway. I was Catholic. Plus, I wanted my baby. Dad wanted me to give it up for adoption.

He took me to the local parish priest. I sat there, across from the stern-faced man of God and watched as my father scribbled some words onto a page, then handed his confession over. The priest, after seeing what my father wrote, told me I was too young to have a child and that the best thing would be to give my baby up.

I looked the priest straight in the eye and said, "I'm not going to do that. I'm keeping my child."

Dad tried, again, to talk me into giving my child up for adoption. You're too young, Pat. You can't do this to yourself. Give the baby up. You'll both be better off.

I had never disobeyed him before, and the thought that he might disapprove of me broke my already fractured heart, yet I stood my ground. With tears streaming down my face I told him, *I'm never giving up my child.*

Once Dad knew he wasn't able to convince me, the next step was to get Bert to marry me. Dad asked Claire to go with him to see Bert and his parents. I wasn't invited, which meant Claire would act as his translator.

I was well aware that my fate was being decided without me, but I was resigned. The only choice that really mattered to me, I'd already made. I was keeping my baby.

Later, Claire told me what transpired:

After she and Dad showed up unannounced on the Young family doorstep and Mr. and Mrs. Young ushered them inside, Dad's fingers flew and Claire acted as his mouthpiece.

She told the family I was pregnant and that my father wanted Bert to marry me. Bert informed Dad that he didn't want to marry me and said that Dad couldn't make him, to which my father replied, *If you don't marry my daughter, I will have to kill you.*

Dad, with his height and strength, could be intimidating.

Bert tried not to telegraph his fear. He folded his arms across his chest. "If you do that, you'll go to jail."

I might be in jail, Dad acknowledged. But you'll be dead.

Bert and I were married within two weeks.

8   Motherhood

When Zach was born, I was seventeen. I'd told myself, prior to his arrival, that the slide into motherhood would be effortless. I was used to cooking, cleaning, and caring for others. When I was in labor, all the attending staff were making a fuss about how young I was. That was when it dawned on me that I was a child who'd assumed responsibility for raising a child.

Once I became a mother – officially – I went into shock. Parenting my siblings Margot and Bernard, and to some extent Barbara, was a whole different dynamic than raising my own baby boy. When I brought Zach home from the hospital, I couldn't stop staring at him. It was surreal. He was so beautiful and I couldn't understand how someone like me could have such a beautiful baby.

As we got older and each of us became more capable of reflection, Zach and I would often talk about how we were two kids growing up together.

I've apologized – profusely – for not giving him better tools for navigating life, and he's forgiven me repeatedly. He understands better than I do – even with all my years of therapy and recovery – that you can't teach skills you haven't yet acquired.

Considering my low self-perception, I'm a little surprised I was able to do as well as I did. Especially since, for most of those early years, Zach and I were all alone.

I didn't get to know my first husband until after we were already married. Our early dating days had been all about his conquest. And after I got pregnant and Dad coerced him into marriage, we continued to live separately – Bert with his parents and me with my mom and siblings.

Within six months of Zach's birth, Bert joined the army. He spent two years in the service, most of those years stationed in Germany. During his time overseas, we kept up a constant communication via letters and pictures. Then, when he returned, we tried to make the best of things. We rented a small one-bedroom apartment in Washington Heights and began our life together.

We lasted less than a year.

Bert was highly critical of me and was a terrible father to Zach. He believed if you criticized someone enough, they'd do better. I couldn't have that kind of negativity around my son. I think he was relieved when I asked him to leave. He'd never wanted Zach or me to begin with. He just hadn't wanted Dad to kill him.

Bert moved out and Mom and my three siblings moved in. Despite the tiny, cramped apartment and our ongoing financial woes, I was a lot happier, and Zach was surrounded by people who adored him. I was glad to give him that.

One of my many regrets was exposing my child to a punitive father when he was between the age of three and four years. Zach was shy and sensitive and Bert reminded me of Dad's mother, and Mom's father. Although shame and low self-esteem had made it nearly impossible for me to advocate for myself, I was fiercely protective of those I loved. I banished Bert for Zach's sake, but it was the beginning of an end to the cycles of abuse I was exposed to as a child. And I have my first son to thank for that.

9 Dennis

It wasn't long after Bert's and my separation that I started dating the man who would become my second husband: Dennis Hart.

Ironically, Dennis was best friends with Bert's brother, Joe. But Dennis wasn't like Bert at all.

He made it clear that he liked me, not as an object to be acquired, but as a person. In fact, until my divorce from Bert became finalized, Dennis and I didn't act on our attraction. He was interested in me for more than sex. It was nice to have a supportive man in my life. One with ambition who was making something of himself. When we first became involved, Dennis was still in college with his eye on medicine. He was originally going for engineering, but a close family friend influenced him to go into medicine. That made me admire him even more. I liked the idea of a man who could help people. There was so much I liked about Dennis. He was intelligent and humorous, and, although he wasn't very attractive, his attraction to me sent me spilling head-over-heels for him.

Dennis encouraged me to improve myself – to read and learn and, most of all, to get my GED. He introduced me to many of the great authors, Steinbeck, Wolf, Christie, Dostoyevsky and others, all of whom I read voraciously. When I told him about my desire to be a secretary, he didn't laugh, as I feared he might. He said he believed in me.

Dennis was a huge support, too, in obtaining my divorce. He arranged for me to meet with a lawyer and even paid to accelerate the proceedings. A New York divorce would've been slow, so, in 1958, I flew to Mexico.

Juarez, Mexico was a well-known spot for quick, legal divorces. Dennis brought me to and from the airport. I'd never flown anywhere before – I'd hardly ever been out of New York City – and I was overwhelmed and in awe at the experience of foreign travel. I couldn't sleep a wink, despite the late hour. I stayed awake the whole flight and, as we landed in Mexico, I saw the sunrise.

It was beautiful.

I didn't know what to make of the dusty, unpaved streets, or the incomprehensible (to me) language. I found the first English-speaking taxi driver I could and paid him to take me to the address I was given. Luckily, at the lawyer's office, everyone spoke English. Unluckily, I wouldn't be the only divorce he conducted that day. I arrived to find a lobby full of people and the secretary – a caramel-colored woman with long, dark hair – informed me there'd be quite a wait.

"You might want to walk down the street to the food vendors and get something to eat," she advised.

Obedient, even as an adult, I went back outside, to the dusty road, and trekked a few blocks away to a strip of food stalls. There were burritos, empanadas, delicious cheesy things heaped with salsa and guacamole, yet I was too afraid to order anything other than a hamburger. Still, as I bit into a familiar-tasting beef patty, life felt far from familiar. I felt like such a big girl – traveling on my own to *Mexico*.

The whole experience only took a day. I returned that night, my signed and notarized papers clutched tightly to my chest, and Dennis picked me up from the airport.

"It's done!" I told him.

He leaned over and kissed me, for the first time.

Finally, Dennis, Zach and I were officially free of Bert!

In 1960, while living in upper Manhattan with Zach six years-old, Dennis and I got married. The thing that really won my heart, as far as Dennis was concerned, was the way he and Zach felt about each other.

Dennis adored Zach so much that he legally adopted him. They were inseparable. Dennis taught Zach how to ride a bike, to play baseball, and to defend himself against bullies. I'd sometimes say that Dennis was closer to Zach than he was to me. Barbara loved Dennis too. She was always visiting us – our closeness hadn't abated with age – and the two of them, my sister and my husband, would joke and laugh. They were as close as siblings. Until the betrayal.

Although Barbara had married her husband, Philip, when she was in her early twenties, and they eventually had three kids together, I thought she may have had a teensy crush on Dennis, but Barbara was no Aunt Juline. Her loyalty was always to me.

It was Dennis who couldn't be trusted.

By the time Zach was nine, Dennis and I realized we didn't want him to be an only child. With Dennis's busy routine and moonlighting at other hospitals for extra money, it wasn't as easy to conceive, but after about a year, I got pregnant.

We were overjoyed!

When Edward was born, in 1965, I was twenty-eight-years-old.

From the outset, I was a different mother. I had eleven years to build some confidence and maturity as a parent.

Because Dennis was a medical resident at the time, I had the benefit of professional courtesy. I spent a week in Flower Fifth Avenue Hospital in Manhattan and we weren't charged a dime by the hospital or the obstetrician. One of the things I recall that took place in the delivery room was my dear doctor, Dr. Donnenfeld, who was also Barbara's OB/GYN, trying to distract me by asking "Who is older, you or Barbara?"

I shocked him – and myself – by responding very loudly, "You know damn well I'm older than Barbara!!"

I wasn't fearful with Edward, like I was with Greg. I was fulfilled. It seemed perfect to have two sons. And Zach loved his little brother! Unfortunately, my sense of fulfillment soon became clouded.

Dennis's behavior became radically different shortly after Edward's birth. I suspected him of having an affair. I knew the signs. Had witnessed them in my own father. He was distant, distracted, and wouldn't make time for me and the boys anymore. It turns out I was right, he was indeed involved with a nurse.

Every time I tried to talk to him about it, he denied it vehemently. The infidelity, painful as it was, hurt me less than the awareness that the man I loved wasn't telling me the truth. One evening, when Edward was about six months old, I went to pick Dennis up from where he was working. While I waited, with Edward in tow, I saw a list of names and phone numbers. Dennis's name was there, but the number listed was not our phone number, it was his girlfriend's. I finally had my proof and Dennis and I began the long and difficult process of ending what was once such a promising beginning.

10 Goodbye, Dennis

The Christmas after Dennis and I separated, a large box was delivered to my apartment. The UPS deliverer didn't know that Dr. Hart was no longer living there. He thought he was being helpful by bringing the box to my place when the nearby office of Dr. Meyers, where Dennis sometimes worked, was closed for the day.

I opened the box. Inside was a little black coat in a size much smaller than I wear. It was for Dennis's new girlfriend.

When I called him to come get it, he had the decency to be embarrassed. "I'm sorry, Pat," he said. Shortly thereafter, he was at the apartment door. "I never meant to hurt you."

I shoved the box into his chest. "It's too late."

Then, I closed the door.

When I told my friend Terry, who lived in our building, what had gone on between Dennis and me, she said I should have torn the present into pieces. I told her that, as betrayed as I felt, I would not stoop that low.

"Oh I would," she replied, and as big as the ache in my heart was, I felt momentarily better.

I'd given up everything out of love for Dennis. When he was still in medical school, he'd applied to what was then known as New Rochelle Hospital for his internship. As part of his compensation, we were given a two-bedroom apartment in a development in downtown New Rochelle, New York. To me, a New York City girl, moving to New Rochelle was the equivalent of moving "to the sticks." I actually had to learn to drive, as did Dennis. We went from being subway and bus commuters to being suburban.

And I had to live farther away from Barbara than I'd ever lived before. I made all these sacrifices not knowing that it would be wonderful for Zach, and later Edward. My sons grew up having access to tennis courts, baseball fields, etc. I hadn't known leaving the life and home I knew would turn out to be a blessing. All I knew was that Dennis and I had built a life together, one I was committed to. Too bad he hadn't been committed to me.

I pushed down my resentment – sure, sometimes with food and alcohol, but I shoved it down nonetheless. For my sons' sake, I couldn't afford to hate their father. I wanted them to remain close with Dennis. Zach, especially. He may not have been Dennis's son, biologically, but Dennis was the only father he'd ever known.

The fatal day occurred in the winter of 1968. I refer to it as a "fatal" because it was the turning point in the deterioration of Zach's relationship with Dennis. Dennis's visits to the kids had become so erratic and Zach had not seen his father in weeks.

Dennis was going to take Zach skiing. Zach was so excited, as they hadn't seen each other for a few weeks, and I was excited for him. I helped Zach pack all his belongings and waved as he and his father drove away.

When Dennis and Zach were halfway to Dennis's new apartment in Mount Vernon, New York, Dennis said "Oh, by the way, some friends are coming with us."

But there were no "friends." There was only one "friend" – a female. Zach was so upset. He'd been expecting a weekend of father-and-son fun time. I received a phone call that night after they arrived at Jay Peak, Vermont.

"What's wrong?" I asked when I heard my son's voice. He'd been elated earlier, but now sounded devastated. Zach was beyond upset, as he'd been expecting a weekend of father-and-son fun time.

Zach begged to come home because he was so uncomfortable. His father was a different person around the new woman in his life. Although I didn't go to him, I instructed Zach to ask his dad to either bring him home ASAP or put him on a bus. Dennis waited until the morning, then drove him home.

That one experience of being around Dennis and his new girlfriend profoundly affected Zach. He was down in the dumps for several days and the deterioration of his school work and social activities soon followed.

I had already accepted the fact that my husband was involved with another woman, had started divorce proceedings and served Dennis with papers. He begged me not to proceed, but I was fed up with the lies, the no-shows with the kids, and the broken commitments. I could accept the loss of my husband, but Zach lost his hero.

He was entitled to better.

I felt as if, in some ways, I was bearing witness to what went on with Dad and Aunt Juline. The new woman in Dennis's life – who would eventually become his wife, just as Aunt Juline would become Dad's after Mom died – influenced his attitudes and actions. She steered him toward herself, away from his sons. Strangely enough, I never blamed Dad as much as I blamed Dennis. And, even though I resented Aunt Juline and never referred to her as my stepmom after she and Dad were married (I always called her Aunt Juline), I loved her.

I disliked Dennis's wife, and the hold she had on the man who'd once been my friend and champion. The man who was still my sons' father.

Dennis and his wife moved to Massachusetts, leaving Zach and Edward with me in New Rochelle. I tried to keep the lines of contact and communication open. My boys deserved a male role model in their lives. They shouldn't suffer because the adults in their lives weren't equipped for healthy, mutual relationships. When Edward was four or five, he flew by himself to Boston. It was only an hour flight and he got to sit up front so the stewardess (they called them stewardesses then) could keep an eye on him. He really thought he was something! He was overjoyed. He was going to see his dad!

It was not until much later that I learned that, during the visit, Dennis hardly ever saw Edward – he hadn't prioritized the visit and was out of the house, working, while Edward was left at home with the new woman in his life, a woman Edward didn't even know. Dennis's wife was not nice to either of my sons. Zach once spent two months with his and Edward's dad and the stepmother and saw first-hand that the woman was not a nice person. He also reported that she had a drinking problem. Dennis as well. I knew that already, considering we had once drunk together.

Then followed the years of no communication, no birthday cards and no Christmas presents. Zach grew disenchanted and, I was pretty sure, gave up hope on the father he'd once worshipped. Edward still believed in Dennis. He still had hope.

When Edward was about thirteen years old, he was part of the Youth Group at our church, St. Catherine of Siena and became close to one of the church's youth ministers. The youth minister, a wonderful, savvy woman, told Edward she would take him to Massachusetts to see his dad, if Edward would arrange it.

At this point, Edward had not seen his dad in probably close to five years. When Edward called his father, Dennis sounded reluctant, but said he could meet him.

I don't think Edward could sleep for two days due to his excitement.

As agreed, our youth minister arranged to take Edward to Massachusetts, just outside of Boston, and she set a time to meet him later to bring him home. Edward had been looking forward for time alone with a man he thought loved him, a man who still had his heart. But instead of forging a connection, Dennis took the opportunity with Edward to regale him with stories about his new kids. Dennis and his second wife had had two boys in succession and Dennis was a proud papa, bursting with stories about his second set of sons and how happy he and his new family were together. He went on and on about their tennis club membership and all the things they did together. (Dennis was always an avid tennis player and ironically, so are Zach and Edward). Meanwhile, his child support payments were so far behind. It was an empty gesture, indeed, when, at the end of the visit, Dennis handed Edward $50 and patted him on the back as a parting farewell. That was the last time Edward saw his father.

I finally sued Dennis in the fall of 1979 – almost ten years after the divorce – to collect what was rightfully my sons', I had to go to Boston. When Dennis saw me, his face lit up and he came forward to embrace me, but his attorney stopped him. I'd never have let him touch me. I was so overcome with rage, not about his infidelity, but about the fact that he had failed to provide for our two boys. In those days, divorced women didn't return to their maiden names, but even if they had, despite my animosity toward the man who'd once inspired and adored me, I wouldn't have gone back to my maiden name. I wanted to share the same name as my sons. They were Harts; I wanted to remain one too.

The outcome of the suit was nominal, with a big chunk going to the attorneys, but standing up for my children felt essential. They deserved a better father than the one Dennis turned out to be.

I regret to say that my former husband has left me with more unpleasant memories than good ones. Dennis loved our sons, I feel sure, yet he followed the advice of a wife who wanted to erase all traces of me and my boys from Dennis's life and memory.

When Dennis died in 2004, the boys were never notified of his death. We found out by accident through my daughter-in-law Audrey, Edward's wife, who was working at the Sheraton Hotel in Stamford, CT. She met someone who recognized our last name and told her a man he knew in Massachusetts (Dr. Hart) had recently died. Audrey obtained a copy of Dennis's obituary and there wasn't a single mention of his two sons in Connecticut.

It cut them like a knife. Zach and Edward were fifty- and forty-years-old at the time

I couldn't let the slight stand, so I sent Dennis's wife a card. After extending my sympathy and condolences, I told her it was a shame that Dennis's sons weren't notified of his passing.

If you're concerned my boys might go after Dennis's estate, you're sadly mistaken, I wrote. The only thing they've ever wanted from their father was a relationship.

11

Neil

In the summer of 1970, approximately two years after my divorce from Dennis, I was working as a secretary for an electrical engineering company in Port Chester, New York, an easy commute from where the boys and I were living in New Rochelle. One day, as I was returning from my lunch break – I saw a tall, attractive man in a pinstriped suit and tie outside the office building where I worked.

As I walked toward the entrance, I sensed the man looking at me and a feeling I'd never felt before crept up my body. I almost tripped and fell. I couldn't get to my desk fast enough. Couldn't escape the watchful eye of the stranger who was undressing me with his gaze.

Unfortunately, or fortunately, there would be no escaping Neil Terranova. A little later that same afternoon, my boss walked into my reception area accompanied by the handsome man in the suit.

"This is Neil Terranova," he said. "He'll be spending quite a bit of time in the buildings doing renovations."

"Neil, this is Patricia Hart, my secretary."

A few days later, Neil approached me and asked me to lunch. Even though I saw a wedding band on his left ring finger, I accepted. I was still hurting from Dennis's betrayal and its effect on our sons, mostly Zach. Edward was only five at the time, and oblivious to most of what was going on, but Dennis was the only father Zach had ever known, and his moving out and taking up with the new woman in his life, and severing ties with us, devastated my oldest and most sensitive son.

I felt as if I had to fill the role of two parents. What's more, I was sick of being the "good girl" and having nothing but heartbreak to show for it. I was set for a little romance with a man whose presence made me feel like a woman.

I had no intention of developing a serious relationship with anyone, let alone a married man, but I figured that a meaningless fling couldn't hurt.

After a couple of months of eating sandwiches with Neil in his car, we arranged to have a tryst in a lovely suite of offices in a building he had designed and built. I could feel my attraction to him accelerating, and the feeling was definitely mutual. Neil and I rendezvoused as planned and the experience was everything

I'd wanted; only, it left me wanting more. Neil too. Unlike Bert, who'd gotten what he wanted then attempted to dispense with me, Neil's affection increased after we were intimate.

He hired me as his office assistant – and let his current assistant go with a huge severance package – so he and I could be lovers in and out of the office. Immediately, a playful and near-constant seduction ensued. Nothing went on during the business day, but once in a while I would write out a pink message slip TO: NAT (his initials) FROM: PMH (mine) and the message portion would read *Wanna fool around?*

Neil had unleashed an entirely different side of me and me in him. We alternated between making each other laugh and making each other... Well, things that still make the good Catholic girl inside of me blush.

Neil and I carried on for about a year. We gave each other what we needed – a little fun in the midst of hard, duty-bound lives. I never permitted myself to think about his wife. After all, my mother and I had both been betrayed by our respective husbands and the last thing I'd have wanted was to wreck someone else's home. I saw what Neil and I had as a temporary diversion. Some harmless, inconsequential fun.

Every Saturday morning, while Edward and Zach stayed with friends, Neil would pick me up early and we'd spend the day together, mostly going into New York City on shopping sprees. He was very generous with me, buying me little gifts and taking me to lunch. I felt cherished and adored. And content. Then, early one Monday morning, Neil told me his wife had accused him of having an affair. He hadn't denied it.

When I found that out, I went into the office and cleaned out my belongings.

I cannot continue to be "the other woman," I wrote on a yellow notepad, which I left on my desk. I should've told Neil directly, but I'd grown up in an environment of nonverbal confrontation, where issues were signed or scribbled, never spoken.

After quitting both roles – secretary and mistress – I changed my home phone number and deliberately kept the new number unlisted.

"Do not, under any circumstances, give my number to Neil," I instructed my friends and family.

True to my sister Barbara's nature, when Neil called her and asked for my number, she caved. Barbara knew how much I cared for Neil – knew even better than me, in fact, since I was still trying to convince myself I'd be okay without him. Neil told her he was leaving his wife, and she broke down and gave my new number to him. He called me from a hotel to tell me he loved me and was leaving her. He could've shown up at my apartment, but I think he opted to call because he could've tolerated me hanging up, but couldn't have endured a slammed door in his face. We kept communicating – briefly. But, after three days, Neil returned home. His wife and kids kept calling him and his wife insisted that, if he didn't return, she'd commit suicide.

I told Neil it was not only over, but I didn't ever want to hear from him again,

"It's best that way," I said.

During the next few months, friends kept trying to set me up. I told them all to leave me alone. I couldn't even look at a man. When I was ready to date again, I'd make that decision.

I easily found another job working at Exxon where I had worked for five years in the late fifties and early sixties.

In those days, I was a commodity – intelligent and attractive were the primary assets for a secretary. There were also no laws against sexual harassment. When the Exxon executives, all of whom were married, hit on me, I felt affirmed rather than offended. Nevertheless, when asked to go to dinner, or lunch, my response was always the same: "Are you going to bring your wife?"

I worked for Exxon for nearly a year. Then, I went back to work for Neil.

Three months after starting my new job, I received a letter from him. He had moved out of his house into a motel and was remodeling the cottage apartment on the property he owned to move into after renovations were finished. He said he could no longer live with his family whether I returned to him or not. He also said that, if I chose not to ever see him again, he would respect my decision.

I still have the letter.

What I loved most about Neil was his respect and adoration for me. He was my rock and we each contributed toward the relationship in different ways. We learned from each other.

Neil's brother Fred was gay and Neil couldn't seem to understand or accept that. I sat down with him one day and we spoke at length about his brother's orientation. I helped him to realize it was not a choice and no matter how many times he asked Fred "Don't you want to feel the body of a woman near you?" Fred's reply would always be "I do not!" He thanked me many times for helping him to come to terms with his brother's sexuality, so he could once again become close to his brother.

Neil taught me to play golf. It was so much fun. He belonged to a country club and during the summer we would play in tournaments with our couple friends.

Neil also loved to dance! He helped me to overcome my self-consciousness with dancing. Our almost-ten-year relationship began with a lot of passion. But it quickly morphed into more.

Neil gave me a new lease on life. He even gave me a new name! Before we got together, everyone had always referred to me as Pat, Patty (which I hated), or Patricia. But a year before

Neil died of a heart attack, we were at the country club, looking through the member directory and I came upon the names of actor George C. Scott and his famous wife, Trish Vanderveen.

"I love that name!" I exclaimed.

Neil wrapped an arm around my waist and declared, "From now on, I'm gonna call you "Trish the dish.""

And he did.

Not too long after he passed, I was at a 12-Step convention and mentioned to my dear friend Maisie, who'd come with me, that I missed Neil and how he had called me Trish.

"I wish people would call me that," I said.

Maisie banged, loudly on a table to get everyone's attention and, once all heads had swiveled toward her, she proclaimed "Hear ye, hear ye! From this day forth, this woman will be known as Trish."

My new nickname is part of Neil's legacy of love, but it's far from the only enduring gift he gave me. It was through Neil that I realized how much Dad cared for me. I once took Neil to meet Dad and Aunt Juline, who was technically my step-mother by that time. As my then-boyfriend, later-fiancé, watched me sign, my fingers flying, my face alight with animation, he looked on in wondrous awe.

I think he's impressed by us, I signed to Dad.

He should be impressed by you, Dad signed back. Does he know how proficient you are?

The man of few compliments had given me one, and I tucked it into my heart, where it acted as a salve upon old scars.

12 Loss

On the afternoon of March 11, 1976, Margot called me to say she had bad news: Daddy died in his sleep. I thought I was hearing things.

"What? No!"

With tears in my eyes, I left my job working with Neil, and drove to the Bronx.

Dad had been diagnosed with cancer of the larynx a few years before he died. My sisters and I (we called ourselves the Three Musketeers) had assisted him during his doctor visits and radiation treatments. I recall one visit when the doctor advised us that Dad would have to have his larynx removed. Dad looked so vulnerable. He'd always been a big, brave man. Now, he was a shadow of his former self and I ached with my own impotence in the face of his disease.

I understood how heartbroken he was. The doctor didn't.

After giving us the details, she said, "At least your father is deaf and his voice won't be a great loss."

I proceeded to let her know in no uncertain terms that our father may have been deaf, but he had a voice! Perhaps one that no one outside our family could understand, but we could. He called us each by name in his own inimitable voice. We had a language that was ours and the loss would be profoundly felt, indeed.

I reached out and took Dad's hand. Later, when we were away from the insensitive doctor, I told him, *I wish you'd stop drinking, Dad. I don't want to lose you.*

He couldn't promise me he'd stop – he was too addicted. But he cried. I was in my late thirties and I'd only ever seen him cry once before, when Mom died.

The last time I saw my mother alive was in 1964, on Thanksgiving Day, at her apartment. The following Saturday, Margot called to say Mom was not doing well. She asked for Dennis, who was still my husband then, and was also a doctor, to come see her.

When Dennis arrived, Mom was sitting on the steps to the apartment building where she, Margot and Bernard lived. She was struggling to breathe. My brother-in-law Philip was there as well. Margot and Bernard were so frightened they'd disappeared off to the side of the house where they looked on, terrified, but did nothing. Mom seemed relieved to see Dennis and she reached out for his hand, then slipped, peacefully away.

Dennis tried to resuscitate her, but she was gone. She died of pulmonary edema. He didn't return to our home until 2:30 a.m. I was sitting on the sofa when he came in and, as soon as I saw his face, I knew.

Losing my mother was an out-of-body experience. She was only forty-nine and I was twenty-eight. I'd expected to have more time with her. More than that, being the oldest of my siblings, I had to put on a brave front. Barbara was seven months pregnant with my niece Carolyn, Margot was eighteen and Bernard was fifteen.

In the aftermath of mom's death, I recall feeling a near constant sense of emptiness. I had no idea how to survive a loss. The way I'd been conditioned to get through life was to get over things quickly and not show any signs of "weakness."

Dennis was of no help. Although he was a trained medical professional, he'd never lost anyone close to him. His father had died years earlier, but they'd had a distant relationship. Mom had been the only person in my life who consistently admired and adored me. Still, I cut myself off from emotion and shoved it down, with food and alcohol. Then, soon after, I got pregnant and was so consumed with that, and work, and raising Zach, that I didn't have time to think about losing Mom.

It was not until Edward was born the following October of 1965 that my suppressed sadness came up – and out. I cried for two weeks straight.

13 Goodbye, Barbara

Icouldn't imagine an existence without Barbara. When we were growing up in the Heights, we had a three-block walk to school and Barbara would always hook her arm into mine and pull me close. On freezing winter days, since we couldn't afford gloves, we would pull our coat sleeves all the way down to cover our hands. Then, arm-in-arm, we would face the cold together.

Barbara got scarlet fever when I was three. After the ambulance came to take her away, I sat in a rocking chair for hours – huddled beneath a blanket – terrified and vigilant. I worried I would lose my sister and I knew I needed her to survive.

Barbara needed me too. She and Philip had split up decades earlier, then, after their divorce, they'd fallen in love again, but he'd died before they could reconcile.

Through the men and marriages, the births of our respective children, the triumphs and tribulations, Barbara and I had remained everything to one another.

She was diagnosed with liver cancer in the late 1980s. She spent decades being poked, prodded, tested and retested, before finally succumbing in 2013. My reaction to her death was unexpected. All I felt was relief.

Barbara had been my friend, my confidant, my support, my ally, and my advocate. Witnessing the deterioration, first of her body and later her mind, my love fed off of itself until it filled all of me, the way the cancer had filled her.

The last two years of my sister's illness were very difficult for me. (They were for everyone!) Barbara lost so much weight she looked like a skeleton and was so unsteady on her feet that she needed to lean up against walls in order to stay standing. She prayed constantly to be cured. She didn't mind dying, she told me, but she didn't want to leave her kids or her eleven grandchildren, all of whom adored her.

Barbara was living with her youngest – my niece – who is a registered nurse. We all derived a great deal of comfort knowing she was in good hands. Although Chelsea lived in Monroe, New York, farther away from me than the Bronx, I visited her as often as I could. In Barbara's last months, I found it more and more difficult to see her in pain. I would sit in her room, while she read or watched TV, and pray for an end to her pain.

But it wasn't all doom and gloom. True to form, Barbara knew how to make me laugh.

She'd close her eyes and feign sleep and I'd go to turn off the TV, so she could rest in silence, and she'd pop open her eyelids and bark "Don't turn it off, I'm watching it!"

Until Barbara died, I'd never known a day without her. Whether in person or on the phone, we spoke from the day our parents brought her home until the day she took her last breath. I miss my sister more than words can say – the silly things we would laugh about – but I always cared more about her than about myself, so I'm glad she's at peace.

14 Recovery

I had my first drink when I was fifteen. I didn't care for the taste of it but I liked the effect. Alcohol lowered by inhibitions and let me forget my responsibilities. So, I'd sip a Manhattan or a Pink Lady (the drinks of the era) and be grateful for the inevitable relief.

Drinking was an occasional thing in the beginning. As soon as I got pregnant with Zach, I stopped – cold turkey. Then, after he was born, I was too busy taking care of him and earning a living to support Mom and my siblings to give in to the temptation to imbibe.

It wasn't until I met Dennis, who I later came to realize was an alcoholic, that I upped my intake and my tolerance. He told me to forget about "those sissy drinks" and introduced me to Scotch. I had to acquire a taste for Scotch, but it didn't take long!

When I drank, I was a different person. I lost my insecurity and shyness and became downright brazen. I also did a lot of things I wasn't proud of.

Many times, after a bout of drinking, I would not recall how I drove home without getting into an accident. When Dennis and I were still engaged, I slept with someone I met at my company's Christmas party. At another party, I got on stage and did an imitation of Carol Channing. Under the influence of alcohol, I would say and do things I would've never said or done sober.

Over the years, my drinking ebbed and flowed. Once I started, it was hard to stop. I was genetically predisposed to addiction, due to my family history.

But it was after Neil died that my drinking spiraled out of control. I drank alone and hid it from my son Edward, who was still living at home. Hiding wine under my bed and getting drunk while alone, then waking up hungover in the morning, I felt like a fraud. That was also what led me to seek sobriety – the feeling of dishonesty. Living a lie was excruciating.

When I first began attending 12-step meetings, I felt out of place. I would envy people who shared "drunkalogs" and had spectacular stories because they had no illusion of functioning through addiction. They were "low-bottom" drunks. Their only hope was sobriety. Then, one day, I realized how fortunate I was to have experienced a "high bottom." I also realized that my drinking, too, had serious consequences – not only for me but for my sons. When Zach was about eight-tears-old, I got so drunk at a bon voyage party for my cousin that I could hardly walk. The car we were all piled into had to repeatedly stop so I could get out and throw up. I was left with a hangover that lasted three days. Zach deserved a better example than that. AA taught me that the only person who could determine whether or not I am alcoholic is me. And, while I may have been functional, my life was far from fulfilled. I kept trying to obliterate pain, kept trying to erase shame. I didn't know that I could move through it and acquire true joy, serenity and peace. How could I? In addition to the genetic predisposition, I'd been conditioned toward self-obliteration.

My eating disorder existed way before my drinking. In fact, my addiction to sugar was the prominent reason I went into Overeaters Anonymous. People think *Food can't be an addiction. You need it to live.* But the insanity I suffered around wanting to consume sugar led me to a feeling of desperation.

As of February 2019, I am, by the grace of God, sober from alcohol for thirty-three years. Yet, when the drinking lessened, my sugar addiction went through the roof! It wasn't long – a month, but that was all it took – before I knew I had to let go of sugar too. I'd given up smoking in 1981, and that was difficult, but giving up sugar was harder than that and alcohol combined.

As of March 2019 I have abstained from eating refined sugar (cookies, cakes, candy and ice cream) for over thirty-three years. Abstaining from my old behaviors with food also includes not eating between meals. It was only when I let go of seeking comfort outside myself from substances that I could confront the true source of my cravings.

All my life, I'd felt like I needed to be "better" than I was. I carried so much shame and self-loathing within me that I didn't know how to function. And there was the incest.

Recovery provided me with the opportunity to review my past with the heart of a lion. I was able to fiercely, and fearlessly, embark on a journey of self-discovery that lasted years – and continues to give shape and substance to my life today. One of the many sayings that I respect is that of Santayana..."Those who do not acknowledge the past are condemned to repeat it." Somehow, viscerally, I knew I needed to break the patterns of my past, but discarding the lessons I'd internalized has been the biggest challenge of my life.

One of my spiritual directors told me that my soul's door was never closed. There was at least a ray of light waiting for me to open the door wider. There is no doubt I have done that.

I treasure my sobriety and abstinence from sugar and the gifts my 12-step programs have brought me. I've become a better woman, better sister, aunt and friend. My recovery is an ongoing process wherein I receive flashes of amazing awareness. I'm also profoundly human. I make mistakes – many mistakes. They keep me humble and therefore teachable. I don't believe I'll ever "arrive," but I hope to remain forever on the "train" of spiritual progress, and to make many, many starts and stops on my journey to eternity.

I developed an even purer love for my parents by working through the issues I had with them and facing my demons head on. I yelled and cried in therapy for years to the point of unravel – only to find the spool of love inside of me could be woven back together. Sure, for several years, I didn't like Dad (or Mom for that matter); but with the assistance to see them for who they were, I left with only gratitude and acceptance toward them and the many gifts they gave me. All those years of being my parents' eyes and ears instilled in me a capacity to see with my ears. In this way, I believe I can hear God's silent whispers in my life. I try to be attuned to different attitudes and perspectives. I have a spirituality that goes far beyond the sin and shame and face-slapping nuns of my youth.

It was not until I was well into recovery and had been going to therapy for several years that I learned that my inner dysfunction also carried with it positive consequences.

Being the "good girl" gave me the groundwork I would later use to overcome my inner adversity. I'd always wanted to do the "right thing." The only problem was that I was never sure what "right thing" would be sufficient to quell the shame. The principles of 12-step recovery offered a roadmap. Working through the twelve-steps, praying, meditating, developing a relationship with a loving Higher Power, following the directions of a kind, accepting sponsor... Gradually, all these things enabled me to rebuild my shattered self-esteem.

One of the many things I learned in the twelve-step meetings was that my addiction and my childhood weren't my fault, but overcoming them was my responsibility.

Growing up with deaf parents was hard. The deaf were considered mentally challenged and, I daresay some even thought deafness was a communicable condition. Most, if not all, deaf men and women were underpaid for their work.

I remember traveling with Barbara and Dad on the trolleys and subways and Dad keeping his signing to a minimum so as not to attract attention.

The deaf community did not have interpreters as they do today. My parents had me and Barbara. As we got older, if Barbara and I were out in public with Mom or Dad, she'd catch people staring at us sideways and demand "What are you looking at?" But I never confronted them. I was too ashamed – not of my parents, exactly, but of feeling different. Out of place.

My parents didn't do a great job of parenting. They didn't have the tools. Today, I recognize that few of us do. Their challenges, however, were more difficult than most. Not only were they young when they had me, they were tasked with surviving in a hearing world, a world that seemed stacked against them.

Yes, my mother parentified me by having me care for her and my siblings and, as a consequence, I lost out on much of my own childhood, but she was depressed and had little to give. My wonderful long-time therapist helped me to reconcile the realities that my mother did the best she could *and* that I deserved better. I grew up ill-equipped to survive in this big, often cruel, world. But that didn't mean I didn't receive tremendous blessings from both my parents.

From my mother I learned about unconditional love. She was utterly accepting of me and all my choices, and the way she forgave and loved her sister showed me the true power of embracing and forgiving others, even if their actions are deplorable. And from my father I learned that the best heroes are the fallen heroes, and I've been able, slowly, to forgive myself for my own shortcomings as a parent.

My gratitude for the incest recovery experience is abounding. It was here that I began to pull the thread of my own ball of yarn of forgiveness. Through prayer, imagery, journaling and a lot of meditation, I was able to start the process of forgiving my grandfather. Hate and shame had kept me a prisoner. It was up to me to break free.

Although it didn't happen quickly – and I know now it wasn't supposed to – I forgave my grandfather. I forgave him for stealing the innocence of a beautiful little girl. I came to learn that he acted out of his own illness, and the awful upbringing he had. One thing my grandfather used to talk about was how he resented his mother for taking him out of school when he was seven. He never learned to read or write. Not even his own name. When he received his checks, he signed them with an "X."

In my meditations, I bravely faced my grandfather and asked him why he'd hurt me. To my surprise, the man I envisioned actually apologized. I felt something deep within shift irrevocably. I knew that he'd hurt me because he was hurting and that I owed it to myself to heal.

One qualification I would like to make, especially for anyone who has experienced any form of sexual abuse, is that I am not advocating forgiveness for everyone. It wasn't even my goal when I set out to reclaim my sense of self. It was a byproduct of working through my pain, shame and anger. And, even when I did forgive, I never condoned (and never will condone) or exonerated my grandfather. I simply let go of the anger that tied me to him.

Years ago, a friend I met in recovery
suggested I begin regularly looking in the mirror
and saying "I love you." At first, it was so difficult I could barely get the words out. In the
early days of beginning the practice, I had a
wall-to-wall mirror in my bathroom. No matter
where I was in the bathroom, I could see
myself... especially when getting out of the
shower. There I was, the full Monty, and I had
to love that? It took a while and eventually as I
got older and the body began to sag, it took
more and more affirmations, but I kept at it and
eventually began to feel something in me shift. It
was a flicker of a flame. The more kindling I
added, the more the flame became a full-blown
fire of self-love.

At the time of this writing, I am eighty-two-
years-old. I'm not exactly happy about that. I
didn't think I'd live this long. Mom died at
forty-nine, Dad at sixty-one. Barbara left this
world at seventy-five. I couldn't have imagined
a world without the three of them until I
reclaimed my own sense of self-worth. Or,
better yet, acquired it. I can't remember ever
having felt I had worth outside of my role as a
caretaker and spokesperson until I entered
recovery. It was there that I realized that I have
a voice of my own, and that God has a purpose
for me.

15   Revisiting Old Memories

As youngsters my parents attended the New York School for the Deaf in upper Manhattan. At some point, the school moved to White Plains, New York.

I'd driven by the huge sign on I-287 going towards the Tappan Zee Bridge many, many times. It read *NEW YORK SCHOOL FOR THE DEAF (NYSD)* in huge, unavoidable letters.

I'd think, sometimes, that it would be nice to go there for a visit, but I didn't act on the impulse. After all, what reason did I have to be there? I'm not deaf, have no school-aged children, and am so long retired that I couldn't show up and ask about a job. I had no pretense for going. No legitimate reason, until 2018.

That fall, I was tasked with hiring an interpreter for a special mass we were having at my church for people with special needs, and I contacted the school for information and resources. It turned out that someone else at my church had already found an interpreter, but during the back-and-forth conversations I'd had with an administrator at NYSD, we'd gotten pretty friendly. The administrator was also the child of deaf parents. Although she is a lot younger than I am, there was a lot of reminiscing on both our parts about what it was like growing up with deaf parents.

"Times have certainly changed!" I observed.

She and I talked about how, just a couple of years earlier (in 2016), a deaf man had won first-place on *Dancing with the Stars*. He, like so many deaf people today had a full-time interpreter at his side. That was not even a remote possibility during my parents' lifetime. I wished my parents were alive to witness Nyle DiMarco accept his trophy. I'm sure being deaf contributed to Dad's alcoholism. He felt a lot of shame and, unfortunately, some of that shame rubbed off on me.

The administrator and I agreed to meet so she could show me around the grounds, including the museum.

When I arrived at the school, I felt simultaneously at home and out of place. To sign after so many years of not doing so was so heartwarming, yet I quickly learned that a lot of my signs were "old school." I was glad to be introduced to some new ones. Part of my visit involved seeing memorabilia from the days my parents attended the school. I glanced into a glass display case and immediately started welling up with tears.

One of the photos was an 18" x 21" picture of my parents in their graduating class of 1935. They looked so young. Mom was so pretty, and Dad was so handsome! They were exactly as I wanted to remember them.

16 Service

In 1990, my parish, St. Catherine of Siena, and the Congregational Church in Old Greenwich, CT held a joint Lenten program in the home of one of the congregants. We met weekly for several weeks and it was there that I heard the hostess mention that she volunteered at a women's prison in Danbury, Connecticut.

This piqued my curiosity.

"What's involved?" I asked.

She told me about how she visited women in prison and I felt a tiny inner tug. I thought of how I'd never reconciled with Claire and, also of how I'd felt internally imprisoned for so long. I imagined I could offer these incarcerated women support and understanding. But I didn't volunteer right away because, despite all the ways in which I'd evolved, I still sometimes let insecurity get the best of me.

Several weeks after the Lenten program was over, I received a call from the same hostess asking if I was interested in joining a group going to Israel. I told her going to Israel was not in the cards, but I asked if she would tell me more about her experience with visiting women in prison. She explained that Prisoner Visitation and Support (PVS) was a national group of people who visited prisoners who didn't get visits for various reasons. The majority of the prisoners were from the New England area which also included New York, New jersey and Pennsylvania. And many of their friends and family lived too far away to come and see them.

That was all I needed to hear. I applied to PVS to be a visitor at the federal prison in Danbury, Connecticut, known as the Federal Correctional Institute (FCI). After I was vetted I needed to get some training which required a trip to the Metropolitan Detention Center in downtown Manhattan. Within a year, our coordinator of visitors asked me if I was ready to transfer to Danbury and I most certainly was!

The prison complex had two facilities – the FCI (Federal Correctional Institute) and the FCC (Federal Correctional Camp) – referred to as simply "The Camp." The FCC housed 1200 male prisoners while the FCC was dedicated to females. The Camp was originally the site of the Watergate detainees and, at the time they were interred, there were eight men – a far cry from the over two hundred female prisoners it came to be.

Visiting the Federal Detention Center in downtown Manhattan was quite an experience.

The women there were awaiting their trials and some of them had been there, languishing for months. Almost everyone had public defenders who served too many people to act expeditiously. Visiting prisoners who were awaiting trial was a very different experience than visiting those serving sentences.

Within months, the men in the facility were replaced by women prisoners. A decision made by the Bureau of Prisons and for reasons only they knew. However, I chose early on to visit the women at the Camp which is a low-security facility in another area of the prison's complex. I hadn't wanted to see the men; my interests lay with helping women.

I visited once a month for 26 years and saw as many as six prisoners a day – each for approximately thirty minutes. I once met Leona Helmsley who, just as expected, attempted to defy the rules even after being locked up. She would ask her peers for favors and services, then refuse to pay them what she'd agreed on.

Leona met her matches, however, in her fellow prisoners. They didn't let her get away with anything. She'd get in line for food and those she'd slighted would refuse to serve her. There would be no special privileges at the Camp, and she was quickly made to get in line.

Although one of PVS's rules was that we were not permitted to ask why someone was in prison, the women usually volunteered the information. They seemed to want to unburden themselves and I found that most of them had been imprisoned for drug-related offenses.

Prior to volunteering there, I'd heard people refer to the Danbury Federal Prison as a "country club" and, although that may have been true when the Watergate guys were there, that had long-since ceased to be the case. Each month, the women would tell me about the faulty plumbing, expired food, and substandard cell conditions.

I loved visiting these women, but I regretted that they had to be patted down before and after every visit. Some of the male corrections officers took advantage of these opportunities, and the women had no defense. They knew that if they filed a complaint, they would become a target for further abuses; so they toughed it out.

During my tenure as a volunteer, at least two women got pregnant from duty officers. The men lost their jobs and benefits, yet the women were left with unwanted babies that were sent to be raised by their families, or given up for adoption. In each of these two cases, these "relationships" were said to be consensual, but I saw them as abuses of power. Still, I imagined the female inmates must've felt sexually stifled. Some of them would even open up to me about it. Others, however, were used to celibacy.

Two of the inmates that I visited throughout the years were Catholic nuns imprisoned for protesting against the United States government. They'd broken into a U.S. nuclear weapons complex, where bombs were stored, and scattered their blood in effigy. These women were amazing and taught more about standing up for faith and values than any of the sisters tasked with instructing Barbara and me at St. Rose of Lima.

After some soul searching, I decided to retire from PVS in 2015. I loved the time I spent there, but I was in my late seventies and I felt like it was time to move on. Nevertheless, the twenty-six years I spent in service changed me in immeasurable ways. I owe a debt of gratitude to PVS and am in awe of all they do in Federal prisons all over the country. Every woman I visited taught me something about myself. By far, the most universal, and most valuable, lesson was that I needed to treasure my freedom. I never take for granted that I can take a hot shower in private, eat in private, watch TV in private...

Epilogue

In 1999 I asked my son Edward if he would accompany me on a trip to the house where I grew up in Washington Heights. I wanted to revisit my childhood home, thinking it might be an opportunity for closure. I was 62 years old and had not been there since I was a teenager. Edward and a friend picked me up on a Saturday afternoon and off we went on a very nostalgic adventure. One of the first things I noticed was the shift in population from the Caucasian/African American blend of my youth to what seemed like 100% Latin American.

When we arrived at the site of what was once my grandparents' house, we encountered instead a huge mound of rubble. Apparently the house was in the midst of being demolished. It was such a shock to see that I had to sit for a few minutes to absorb this loss. I began to cry silently. Edward was upset and I assured him I was okay. I also told him my tears were of joy – all the pain, the sexual abuse, the cold and damp of the rooms, the lack of heat and hot water, my father's betrayal of my mother,

Claire... all of it felt like it was being demolished along with the physical components of 465 West 165th Street.

It was an appropriate finale to my life in that house and to my connection with Washington Heights.

Acknowledgements

There have been many people who were helpful during my journey of writing my memoir and too many to name. The people I do want to acknowledge are: Daralyse Lyons, my editor, who took the "bag of tricks" that I sent her and created the copy that became my life's story. I am indebted to her and her talent for creating.

Grace Halsey who, from the very beginning approximately twelve years ago, encouraged me to write a page at a time and not worry about the order – in other words, let my editor take the responsibility for that. Grace did the first proof of my manuscript in spite of her very busy schedule and, did a second read as well. Grace, your encouragement and support were what got me to keep going on.

Muffie Dunn also read my manuscript and offered so much constructive advice proving to me she is, indeed, a gifted writer herself. You were a gem at a time when I needed strong wisdom and support. Thank you, dear Muffie; you took time out of an unbelievable time of career change and still devoted so much time to getting my book off the ground.

Thank you dear friends; I could not have completed this manuscript without your love, support and creative encouragement.

About the Author

I was born and grew up in New York City. I lived in three of the five boroughs: Manhattan, Brooklyn and Queens. In Washington Heights, Manhattan, there was a concentration of Irish and Italian immigrants, and just around the corner was Harlem with the African American population. As a matter of fact, the street where I lived was all Caucasian on one side and all African American on the other, and if you walked five streets west, you were in the Jewish neighborhood. Until I was in my teens, this mixture prevailed until the Latins started moving in; today, Washington Heights is all Latin. I was fortunate to have been exposed to this diversity, although everyone stayed in his/her specific designated area. My parents were first generation Irish and Italian, and because we lived with our Italian grandparents, our exposure was stronger towards that ethnicity.

I am the child of deaf parents – my father was also an alcoholic, and my mother suffered from depression. We lived with both poverty and a grandfather who was a tyrant too cheap to convert the house we lived in to have heat and hot water. I know full well what it's like to wash my hands and face every morning with cold water and to live in a cold, damp house. We also had no bathroom; a closet in the hallway with a commode and flusher was the extent of our bathroom. I didn't see a tub until I was fourteen and we moved to subsidized housing in Queens. Living in compromise was something my family and I were very familiar with.

When I share my growing-up years with people, they usually find it hard to believe. I'm sure there are many people who also lived without hot water and heat, but probably not in New York City! In addition to these inconveniences, there will probably be many people who identify with having parents who were "different," such as those who are immigrants, which has its own challenges. My hope is for people to see the resilience and see themselves in this book.

It was important for me to memorialize my life, from childhood to adulthood; from being "not enough" to being everything God created me to be. From confusion to clarity. From self-loathing to self-love. The journey was tough but well worth every tear and heartache I experienced to get to where I am today.

I hope readers will see themselves on these pages and recognize the image of hope and strength and be encouraged to forge ahead – especially with recovery. The most fantastic thing I have been given, besides my sons, grand-sons and daughter-in-law, is my sobriety, which was the pivot point to so much more growth and recovery – not possible to name them all!

After a life of responsible living – eldest child, young mother, diligent employee, respected manager – I am loving the life of retirement (after fifty-five years of service to the working world) and pretty much doing what I want, when I want. The first thing I did when I retired, almost nine years ago, was NOT use my alarm clock! I've learned that doing nothing is still doing something, although my doing nothing still involves volunteering at my church and at the hospital, being a sponsor to several women and taking time out to just chill with a good book or a good movie.

I think I'll just continue to do the same...one day at a time!